# THE FOOD DOCTOR DAILY DIET

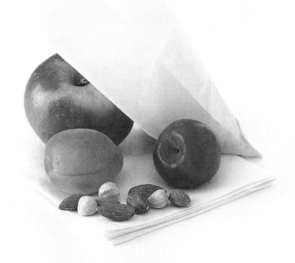

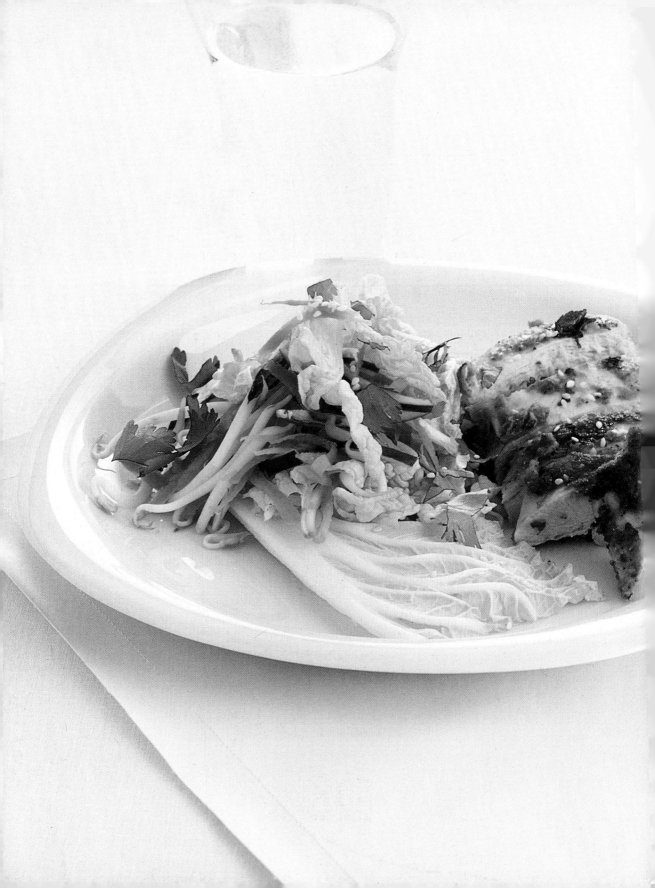

# THE FOOD DOCTOR DAILY DIET

## Ian Marber Dip ION

### Keep in touch and stay in shape

Sign up at **www.dk.com/fooddoctortips** to receive
a monthly email full of encouragement from
Ian Marber, the Food Doctor

For more information on The Food Doctor,
visit **www.thefooddoctor.com**

LONDON, NEW YORK, MELBOURNE, MUNICH, AND DELHI

For my wonderful mother
with thanks, appreciation and love

With special thanks to Rowena Paxton for her truly delicious recipes and to George, Alistair, and Henrietta Paxton for being willing guinea pigs

**Project Editors** Jennifer Lane, Janice Anderson
**Project Designer** Jo Grey
**Senior Art Editor** Rosamund Saunders
**Managing Editor** Stephanie Farrow
**Publishing Manager** Gillian Roberts
**DTP designer** Sonia Charbonnier
**Production Controller** Stuart Masheter
**Art Director** Carole Ash
**Publishing Director** Mary-Clare Jerram
**Food stylist and home economist** Pippin Britz
**Photographer** Sian Irvine
**US Editor** Jennifer Williams
**US Nutrition Consultants** Lisa Hark, PhD, Darwin Deen, MD, MS
**US Recipe Consultant** Wesley Martin
**US Editorial Assistant** John Searcy

**Note to readers:**
Do not attempt the Food Doctor Daily Diet if you are pregnant or under 18. Please consult your doctor first if you have a diagnosed medical condition.

Use either all metric or all imperial measurements. Metric and imperial measurements are not interchangeable so never combine the two.

First American Edition, 2005
2 4 6 8 10 9 7 5 3

Published in the United States
by DK Publishing, Inc.
375 Hudson Street
New York, New York 10014

DK Publishing, Inc. offers special discounts for bulk purchases for sales promotions or premiums. Specific large-quantity needs can be met with special editions, including personalized covers, excerpts of existing guides, and corporate imprints. For more information, contact:
Special Markets Department,
DK Publishing, Inc., 375 Hudson Street,
New York, NY 10014 Fax: 212-689-5254

Cataloging-in-Publication data for this book is available from the Library of Congress.

ISBN 0-7566-0593-8

Color reproduced by Colourscan, Singapore
Printed and bound in Portugal by Printer Portuguesa

Discover more at
**www.dk.com**

# Contents

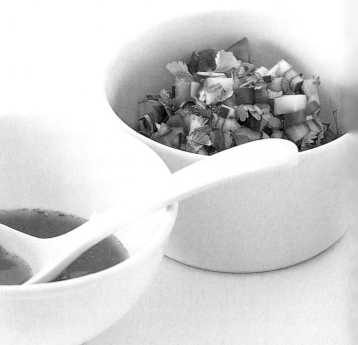

# Everyday eating

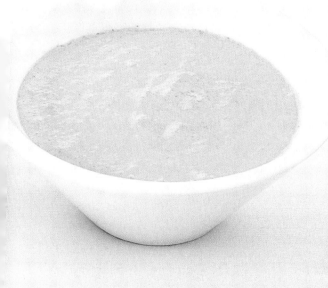

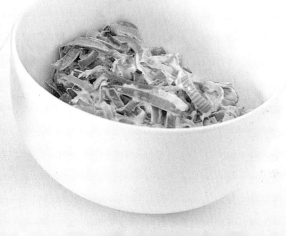

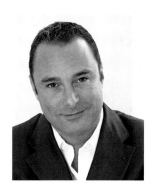

# Introduction

My aim in writing *The Food Doctor Daily Diet* is to show you how easy it can be to lose weight at a sustainable rate, while eating nutritious food and not having to cut out any food groups.

The Food Doctor plan was written after many thousands of hours of working with people who wanted to lose weight. The principles that I believe in are safe, accessible, and easy to incorporate into any lifestyle. I know they work and have witnessed their success time and time again. There are no potentially unhealthy side-effects, and they re-establish the value of proper food in the complicated arena of weight management. The 10 principles (*see pp.12–13*) that form the foundation of my plan are very simple to incorporate into your everyday life, yet so effective.

## A diet for the Real World

So, what is The Food Doctor Daily Diet? Simply a diet you can follow every day without actually feeling as though you're "on a diet" at all— a diet that can work for you whatever your lifestyle. Over a number of years, I have gathered feedback from private clients ranging from regular people to musicians, actors, performers, and models. Each situation was different, and so my diet plan evolved to suit all situations and life-styles, including work, staying at home, and a multitude of careers and life pressures. Whether male or female, single or married, with or without children, this diet is easy to incorporate into your everyday life.

Many of you will have been on very prescriptive diets previously, i.e. those that demand that you eat a specific food in a specific amount. With my diet, it's up to you: the recipes work best with the listed foods, but if you don't like something, then by all means substitute one protein for another, or one complex carbohydrate for another. It's your choice, and it's not magic—just sensible, balanced, non-faddy eating in a way that will encourage safe weight loss without side-effects.

In this book you will find more than 100 delicious recipes that are all diet-friendly (although many could be served at a dinner party without your guests ever guessing that they were eating "diet food" with you). They can be mixed and matched as you choose—I've made some

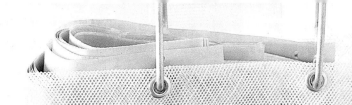

What is **The Food Doctor** plan?
It is based on "fueling up" frequently with
an ideal combination of **protein** and
**complex carbohydrates** at every meal

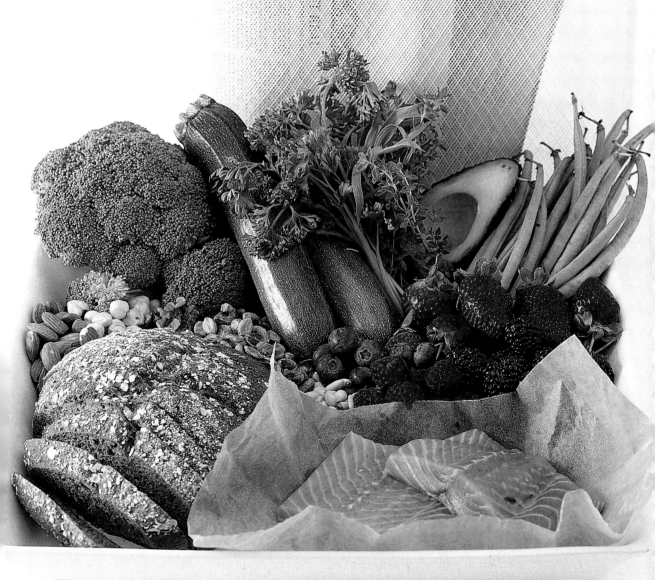

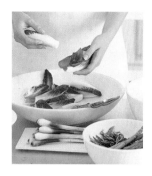

# If you get to a **point** where you **see food** simply as something that will make you **fat or thin**, then **your vision** has become blurred

suggestions, but I hope you will also explore the options for yourself. There are menu ideas to show you how easy it is to combine the food groups according to The Food Doctor plan, and suggestions for how to "tweak" common meal choices to make them that much healthier.

Often this involves taking into account the glycemic index (GI) rating of foods. This is a key factor in The Food Doctor plan, which is geared to fueling your body with a steady flow of energy while minimizing the production of insulin. This is one diet that *doesn't* want you to skip any meals! We examine how food is converted into glucose and the importance of eating in a way that regulates the speed at which that conversion occurs—too rapidly or too slowly will confuse your metabolism and potentially lead to even more weight gain when you return to your "normal" eating patterns.

> "I have been on the diet and can honestly say I haven't looked back! I have lost 56lbs, I feel fabulous and proud of myself. I have never before been on a diet where I have never felt hungry but this is it! "
>
> **Sharon Clifton,** CHICAGO, ILLINOIS

## Time for change

The plan is designed to be practical for those of us that live in the "real world," not in a world of denial, weighing food, starving or bingeing. One reader described my earlier book, *The Food Doctor Diet*, as "A food plan for grown ups" and, while it works for children too, I really relate to that idea. Time seems to be a huge barrier to sensible eating for many people, but with The Food Doctor plan healthy eating becomes a quick, simple option: many of the meal ideas take only minutes to prepare and can actually be quicker than waiting for the microwave to go "ping" with a store-bought prepared meal. Time—and how to make the most of it— is a key element of *The Food Doctor Daily Diet.*

Since I published *The Food Doctor Diet* in 2004, many readers have written to tell me how well it has worked for them. With questions from readers, I have been able to develop the plan and explore new ways of explaining it more clearly for you. This book is the result of that process—a development that expands on the 10 principles outlined in the first book and provides you with even more inspirational ideas on how to incorporate them smoothly and simply into your life. And it doesn't stop here: log on to www.dk.com/fooddoctortips and I'll keep you up-to-date on my latest thoughts and ideas.

One of my key messages concerns how food seems to have become devalued. This is a major factor in why many people have gained weight in the first place, and it's time to revisit the important basics of food. We need re-educating on how to eat, and in turn need to educate children about better eating habits, so that excess weight is not something we pass on to the next generation. The health risks associated with obesity are yet to be really felt and health services worldwide will be further stretched than ever. All because of the food we eat.

"I went on the diet and lost 6lbs, just the boost I needed. I am now trying to stick to the principles and have a lot more energy than I used to have. My husband has joined me in trying to eat more healthily and even the children are enjoying the food. It is so refreshing to have an easy diet to stick to."

Sue Oliver, ALBANY, NEW YORK

## Fads and fashions

Every year there are a plethora of new diet books on the shelves, making claims for instant weight loss. But why are there new diet books every year when nothing has changed in the world of cells in millions of years? The only thing that has changed is the food we eat, along with a food industry hungry for profits and the lack of priority we are now attaching to food. We are all hoping for an easy way to lose weight—something cutting-edge yet easy to do, inexpensive and instant.

But the truth is that there isn't anything new. The body breaks down food in exactly the same way it did when we were living in caves, and no new food has been invented for some time (aside from processed food!) so it seems obvious to me why fad diets cannot work. The problem is that the cutting-edge, well-marketed diet is still a diet, with a beginning, a middle and an end, and so you will "be good," "come off it," or "cheat" and so the cycle begins again.

The Food Doctor plan is one for life, not the short term, and once you understand the principles and incorporate them into your life, you will find that it makes for an easier life, together with true weight loss.

The **Food Doctor** plan aims to provide you with a **steady flow** of **energy**—this is one diet that **doesn't** want you to **skip meals**

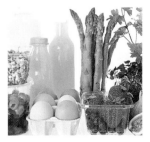

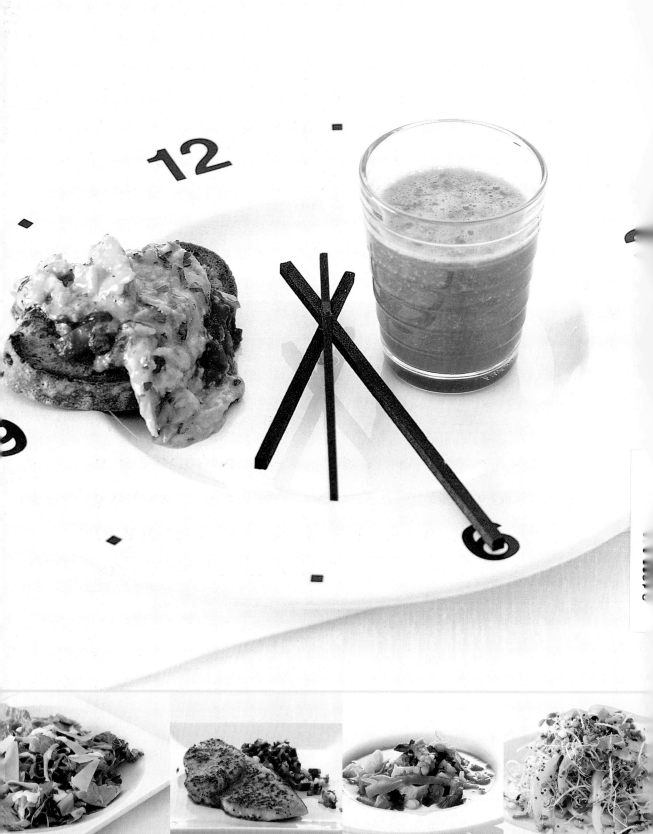

# Principles ¡and science

The 10 Food Doctor principles, my essential guidelines on how to eat, are based on some fascinating concepts. This chapter will show you how poor food choices and long-term or crash dieting can affect your insulin levels and metabolic rate in negative ways. You can then discover how The Food Doctor Daily Diet provides a solution.

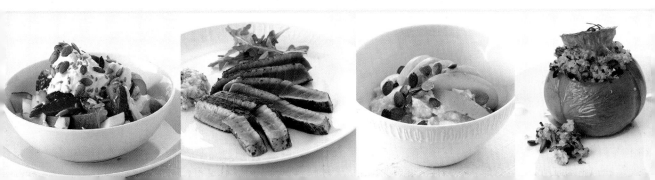

# The 10 principles

These principles are key to my way of eating. They are the "building blocks" for the Daily Diet and have been designed to be simple to remember and straightforward to incorporate into your lifestyle. There are no complicated calorie-counting or points systems. Sticking to the 10 principles is easy and will give you the tools to control your weight, feel healthier, and have a better attitude to food.

PRINCIPLE 1

## Eat protein with complex carbohydrates

Combining these food groups in the correct proportions will ensure that you receive a steady flow of energy, as the body converts foods relatively slowly into glucose. You can then avoid triggering insulin production, therefore minimizing the potential for your body to store food as fat (*see pp.14–19*).

PRINCIPLE 2

## Stay hydrated

It is important to drink plenty of water, preferably at least 3½ pints (1.5 litres) a day—and even more during hot weather, or if you are exercising. Remember that by the time your body tells you that you're thirsty, you are already dehydrated. Limiting your alcohol and salt intake is important too, because these dehydrate the body.

PRINCIPLE 3

## Eat a wide variety of foods

It is easy to get stuck in a routine when shopping: in fact, for 90 percent of the time the majority of us buy just 10 percent of the variety of foods that are actually available to us. Try introducing two new foods to your shopping cart every week.

PRINCIPLE 4

## Fuel up frequently

Eating frequent, small portions of the right foods is a vital part of The Food Doctor plan. Doing this gives you a constant supply of energy throughout the day, avoiding the insulin rollercoaster (*see pp.16–17*) and making hunger, tiredness, and food cravings a thing of the past.

PRINCIPLE 5

# Eat breakfast

Breakfast is essential: eating a balanced breakfast supplies you with the fuel to help maintain energy levels and set your metabolism up for the day. It can be hard to fit it into a busy lifestyle, but taking a few minutes to eat breakfast is fundamental to controlling your weight in the long term.

PRINCIPLE 6

# Avoid sugar

Sugar is present in food in many different forms (*see p.20*), all of which break down into glucose extremely quickly, and all of which therefore contribute to fat production and weight gain. The speed at which sugar converts to blood glucose creates a high, and the resulting low causes hunger.

PRINCIPLE 7

# Exercise is essential

Making progress with The Food Doctor plan does not just depend on changing your attitude toward food. Exercise and healthy eating need to go hand-in-hand in order to get results. However busy your everyday schedule, aim to fit in 30 minutes of exercise three times a week.

PRINCIPLE 8

# Follow the 80:20 rule

It is perfectly normal to "stray" every now and then. If you follow The Food Doctor Daily Diet for at least 80 percent of the time, then you can stray for 20 percent of the time. This means you can enjoy social occasions without feeling guilty, and also escape the boredom and frustration associated with other diet regimens.

PRINCIPLE 9

# Make time to eat

Eating has become rather devalued today. Often it is crammed between more "important" events, and we barely have time to sit down to enjoy our food. Taking time out for a meal is far more beneficial to digestive health, as well as being more satisfying.

PRINCIPLE 10

# Eat fat to lose fat

If you are used to counting calories, you probably view fat as the enemy. However, there are certain essential fats (omega-3 and omega-6) that the body needs to function properly. The key is to eat less saturated fat and to ensure that you consume enough of the essential fats.

# The GI factor

You've probably heard of expressions such as "sugar cravings," "energy slumps," "sugar highs," and "high GI." These relate to the rollercoaster ride of insulin production that many of us put our bodies through by making mistakes in our food choices and dietary habits.

The food you eat is turned by the body into glucose, which is its source of fuel for creating energy. Glucose levels in the body are constantly monitored and kept within strict boundaries by hormones that store glucose when there's too much of it in the blood and release it again when levels are low.

### Insulin and the GI index

Glucose is stored first as glycogen in the muscles and liver, but if glucose levels become high and glycogen stores are full, a hormone called insulin is released to store the excess glucose as fat until the body needs to convert it back to glucose for energy (*see opposite*).

This can have a rollercoaster effect on the body (*see pp.16–17*). In terms of weight loss and gain, it means that if we eat the sort of foods that raise the body's glucose levels too high, or that encourage the body to release too much glucose, then glucose storage speeds up. Since the job of insulin is effectively to encourage the storage of excess glucose, clearly we need to limit the amount of insulin that the body creates in order to discourage the storage of fat. The trick is to choose foods that break down slowly into glucose and therefore avoid

triggering insulin production. However, we should also eat in a manner that does not allow insulin levels to fall too low, since that in turn can also cause serious health problems. Knowing which foods are high in sugar and which ones trigger insulin production is essential to understanding how The Food Doctor plan works. It is why one of my 10 principles advocates fueling up frequently and why I recommend eating foods with low scores on the glycemic index (GI).

A food's GI score is based upon how quickly it converts to glucose in the body. Foods with a high score convert rapidly into glucose (and therefore trigger insulin production), while foods with low scores convert more slowly and are therefore unlikely to raise blood-glucose levels above the insulin threshold.

### What influences insulin production?

A number of foods and other factors have a rapid effect on insulin production, while other foods and factors have very little effect. Watching out for these "highs" and "lows" is key to my plan, but it's very easy to remember and fit into your everyday life. The four main "highs" that raise glucose levels and trigger insulin production, and therefore fat storage, are sugar, simple carbohydrates, stress, and caffeine (*see pp.20–23*). Avoid these factors.

So what are the "lows" that help you maintain steady blood-glucose levels, keeping insulin production at bay and therefore avoiding fat storage in the body?

**Protein** This is quite hard for the body to break down. In other words, it takes longer for the glucose to be extracted, which keeps blood-glucose levels even.

**Complex carbohydrates** Unlike simple carbohydrates, complex carbohydrates are fiber-dense, so it takes longer for the body to break them down into glucose than it does for it to break down simple carbohydrates.

### HOW IS INSULIN LINKED TO FAT?

Minimizing insulin production in the body is an important factor in The Food Doctor plan. To understand why this is, you need to be aware of the relevance of two of its functions in relation to potential weight loss:

- Insulin is a catalyst for the creation of new fat

- Insulin inhibits the breakdown of fat

continued p.18

# How food can turn into fat

If the food you eat is broken down into glucose too rapidly, or if you eat large amounts, then your body will create more glucose than you need. This surplus is stored as glycogen, but glycogen stores have a limit to what they can hold and, when they are full, the excess is stored away as fat.

food is eaten
▼
converts into glucose
▼
enters the blood
▼
reaches every cell
▼
provides fuel
▼ ▼
creates or stored
energy as fat

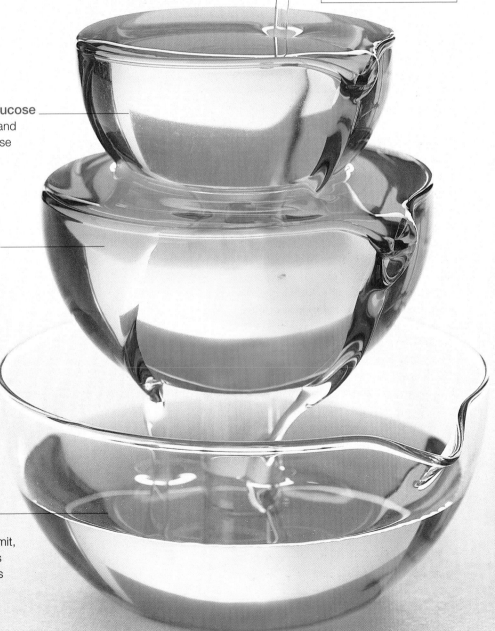

**Food converts to glucose**
Food enters the body and is converted into glucose to provide energy.

**Short-term storage**
If the immediate energy requirements are not high enough to use all the available glucose, or if glucose enters the system too rapidly, the overflow is stored short-term in the liver and muscles in a base of water known as glycogen.

**Excess glucose becomes fat**
If the body's stores of glycogen reach their limit, any overflow of excess glucose still available is stored as fat.

# THE INSULIN ROLLERCOASTER

8am　　9am　　10am　　11am　　12pm　　1pm

The orange line shows the energy and insulin highs and lows of an "average dieter" through the day. The green line of The Food Doctor dieter illustrates how eating the right foods at the right times can maintain energy levels and avoid triggering insulin production.

INSULIN THRESHOLD

The simple carbohydrates, sugar, and caffeine, kick-start your insulin (and therefore fat) production for the day

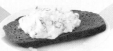

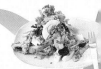

The protein and complex carbohydrates turn slowly into energy, avoiding insulin production

A breakfast of muesli, nuts, and yogurt gives you a good ratio of protein and complex carbohydrates

A mid-morning snack tops up the intake of protein and complex carbohydrates

A combination of protein with simple and complex carbohydrate for lunch provides a steady flow of energy for the afternoon

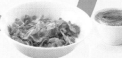

You eat a typical breakfast of cereal and coffee—i.e. simple carbohydrates, sugar, and caffeine

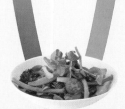

You have a "sensible" lunch, perhaps pasta salad for energy or a salad if you're *really* trying to lose some weight, but there's no protein in your lunch

| KEY | Insulin production | Food Doctor dieter | Average dieter |
|-----|--------------------|--------------------|----------------|

8am　　9am　　10am　　11am　　12pm　　1pm

3pm    4pm    5pm    6pm    7pm    8pm    9pm

As a simple carbohydrate, pasta sends blood-glucose levels quickly back over the insulin threshold, and the lack of protein in your lunch does nothing to slow down this process

A couple of cookies and a dose of caffeine trigger more insulin production

The simple carbohydrates kick in again to send your blood-glucose levels back up into the insulin-producing zone

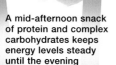

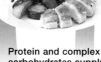

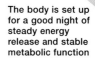

...ergy continues to ...e released evenly ...to the bloodstream, ...elping to keep the ...etabolism steady

A mid-afternoon snack of protein and complex carbohydrates keeps energy levels steady until the evening

Any dip in energy levels is avoided, while the lack of hunger helps you maintain your resolve to make good food choices

Protein and complex carbohydrates supply the right amount of steady energy release to last you through to bed-time

The body is set up for a good night of steady energy release and stable metabolic function

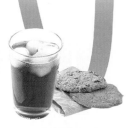

Having had a rapid-burning lunch, you're hungry again by mid-afternoon, so resort to a snack and possibly a caffeine-loaded drink

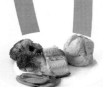

Since your snack was insubstantial, you're hungry again by dinner-time, so you break your diet and eat a large meal of protein and simple carbohydrates

2pm    3pm    4pm    5pm    6pm    7pm    8pm    9pm

**Fiber** This slows the process of glucose extraction from other foods, which discourages rapid or excess glucose production and therefore reduces the need for the body to produce insulin.

To sum up, if you can eat in a way that focuses primarily on these "lows," glucose levels and insulin production will stay low, allowing fat to be released from the fats cells to provide energy rather than encouraging fat to be stored. The 10 principles of The Food Doctor plan are designed to make it easy for you to achieve this.

The Food Doctor plan offers three ideal options for combining food groups that will minimize insulin production and thus minimize potential fat production too (*see box, below right*). There is a fourth, not-so-ideal option, which is to eat complex carbohydrates with fiber but without protein. This is the *least* preferable option because protein is the hardest food group to break down and therefore has the slowest glucose conversion rate, minimizing the risk of triggering insulin production.

## Balancing your protein intake

A diet based largely on protein alone is a popular option, but not one I favor. I have put my plan together so that, when it is properly followed, it will always include the right sort of carbohydrates in each and every meal and snack. I believe that, although we are all different and the requirement for protein in each of us is different, when it comes to safe, consistent weight loss, we should all aim to eat a maximum of 40 percent protein to minimize the risks associated with excess protein intake.

I find that people who follow high-protein diets tend not to eat the recommended five portions per day of fresh fruit and vegetables, which in turn means that their intake of antioxidants will probably be low. These vital substances are linked to reducing the risk of cancer, heart disease, and arthritis. They also help to slow down the aging process, so it's really not a good idea to exclude them from your food intake.

To be fair, most high-protein diets do encourage you to eat some fresh fruit and vegetables at a later stage in the diet, but my long experience with dieters tells me that a large proportion of them do not move on to that later stage. Instead, they stay in the all-fat and all-protein phase, since it requires little thought and there is less room for mistakes. It is at this induction phase that weight loss is most noticeable, but I maintain that this type of eating is not sustainable

and, as such, it is just another diet with a beginning, a middle, and an end. So you "come off" the diet, or "cheat," and the weight reappears. The fact that many people eat this way highlights the sad fact that we choose to ignore what proper dieting can do. This tends to make us look at food only in terms of whether it can make us fat or thin.

Diets that rely on very high levels of protein can have several other potentially harmful effects:

**Fats** The type of protein you can get from eating a high-protein diet is often very high in saturated fats—cheese, for example. Eaten in excess, it may also raise cholesterol levels and thus increase the risk of cardiovascular disease.

**Calcium** Our bodies are designed to keep a balance between acid and alkaline, ensuring that the body's internal environment does not become too acid. Metabolizing protein raises acidity and if there is too much acid, it will be counteracted by the release of calcium from stores, in order to "buffer" the increased acidity. Since most of the calcium in the body is contained in the bones, a very high-protein diet can in the long term lead to decreased bone density. Calcium also has to be excreted and sometimes builds up in the kidneys. Here, it can form stones which, once broken down and passed through the urinary tract, can be excruciatingly painful.

**Fiber shortage** High-protein diets tend to be low in fiber, leading to constipation which in turn increases the risk of colon cancer.

**Sleep problems** There may be another, strange, side-effect of excess protein—on sleep. Proteins contain amino acids, which are used everywhere in the body,

---

### MAKING GOOD CHOICES

In The Food Doctor plan, there are three acceptable ways to combine the food groups :

1. Eat protein with vegetables and starchy complex carbohydrates.

2. Eat protein with vegetables.

3. Eat protein with just starchy complex carbohydrates (although this is the least preferable option with regard to the GI factor).

## A PERFECT COMBINATION

Protein and complex carbohydrates combine a good GI rating with a healthy intake of antioxidants and fiber.

# 40% protein
such as fish, lean meat, or beans

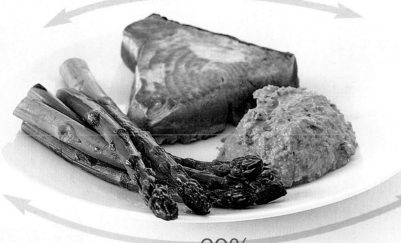

# 60% complex carbohydrates
such as green vegetables with plenty of fiber

including the most vital organ, the brain. Covering the brain is a porous layer of skin called the blood-brain barrier, which acts as a filter, allowing in some substances and protecting the brain from potential toxins. Because the barrier limits overall absorption, amino acids fight with one another for absorption. When carbohydrates are broken down in the body, amino acid levels are suppressed, with the exception of one, tryptophan, which is allowed through. This amino acid is effectively the precursor to sleep so, when excess protein is eaten without carbohydrates, and other amino acid levels are not suppressed, tryptophan cannot pass unhindered into the brain to encourage sleep.

I have heard many people argue that surely all the risks and potential side-effects of excess protein is worth it for the promised weight loss, and surely obesity is just as much of a health risk as any of the other conditions? True, but there are ways of losing weight that do not involve such risks, and I feel that diets very high in protein and fat come with a potential price for you to pay that make them unnecessarily risky.

### The healthy way forward

Understanding the GI factor and learning how to fuel your body in a way that doesn't have negative side-effects, and doesn't distort your attitude to food, is what the Daily Diet is all about. High-protein or low-carbohydrate diets and low-calorie or low-fat diets all bring with them various problems (*see pp.42–43*). The 10 principles of The Food Doctor plan allow you to avoid the pitfalls associated with other common diets. Using these principles, you can establish a healthy eating

# Diets very **rich in protein** come with a potentially **high price** to pay for your **health**

pattern that controls insulin levels, avoids the insulin rollercoaster, and eliminates the danger of disrupting your metabolism (*see pp.24–27*). In this way, it is a plan for life—one that is sustainable enough to last you a lifetime and practical enough to fit into your lifestyle.

# Key insulin triggers

By now you can see how important it is to keep blood-glucose levels as steady as possible. One of the main principles of The Food Doctor plan, "fuel up frequently," is designed to do just this. The amount you eat, how often you eat it, and the ratio of protein to complex carbohydrates in your meals all help to keep blood-glucose levels steady and avoid sending them over the insulin threshold. However, there are other key substances that can act as triggers to promote the release of insulin. Five of these key triggers—sugar, simple carbohydrates, stress, smoking, and caffeine—are explained further here.

The term "insulin trigger" may sound quite alien to you, but these triggers are actually things that you may encounter daily without even thinking about it. Each of these insulin triggers has different characteristics in that some are social, some give you an energy boost, and some are addictive. However, they all involve the same sort of chemical change and reaction in your body when it comes to insulin production.

Insulin allows the body to store fat from the food you eat: Without insulin this process is limited. Avoiding the insulin rollercoaster (*see pp.16–17*) is an important part of the Food Doctor plan, since this will help your body limit the amount of fat stored. Understanding the impact of the key triggers listed here, therefore, is vital to successfully controlling your weight.

---

### THE SCIENCE: ADRENALINE AND GLYCOGEN

Adrenaline is released to assist the body's reaction to a "fight or flight" situation. It is a throwback to our caveman days that can still be triggered by stress situations or stimulants. It has several effects, one of which is to divert blood from "secondary" areas such as the digestive system and pump it to areas primarily involved in fight or flight, such as the muscles, heart, and lungs. Digestion is slowed, hindering the absorption of nutrients and suppressing your appetite. Blood-glucose levels climb rapidly to ensure that muscles have plenty of fuel. When the levels rise too high, insulin is produced (*see pp.14–19*). The rapid rise is followed by a significant drop which triggers a demand for more energy—so you experience hunger.

---

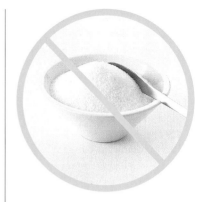

## Sugar

Many years ago I read that as long as a food was fat-free, then it would not contribute to excess weight. So I happily went out and bought lots of sweet, sugary foods that were effectively fat-free, and guess what? Over a short period of time, I gained weight. I believe that fat was given a poor reputation years ago in terms of weight issues. Yet sugar, including honey, has been hiding quietly in the corner hoping that it wouldn't be noticed. It is time to bring the truth about sugar out into the open and recognize its negative role.

### What is sugar?

Sugar lurks in many forms: sucrose, mannitol, glucose, honey, lactose, fructose, sorbitol, corn syrup, malt, malt extract, maltose, rice syrup, rice extract, molasses, golden syrup, and invert sugar are all pseudonyms for sugar. Refined sugar is a simple carbohydrate. In fact, it is almost the epitome of one. As we know, simple carbohydrates are converted from food into glucose much more rapidly than their complex counterparts.

Sugar has only a few bonds to hold it together, making it free of fiber—the fiber that is important for slowing down glucose extraction.

Sugar, therefore, converts quickly into blood glucose, sending you rapidly over the insulin threshold (*see pp.16–17*).

Many of my clients proudly report that instead of eating "regular" chocolate, they eat organic, healthy alternatives. I am pleased about this because it means they are reading food labels and hunting for good alternatives. Sadly, though, however you eat it—organic, raw, brown, or white—it is still sugar. It will still be converted into glucose with alarming speed and have the same effect on blood-glucose levels.

### What about honey?

After all, honey is natural, isn't it? Well, so is sugar—it grows in fields. Honey has acquired a romantic air: we think of bees buzzing around on a warm day collecting nectar and making honey in the hive for the friendly beekeeper to collect. It is true that honey has many beneficial health properties, but it is actually converted into glucose at almost the same speed as sugar. In fact, the GI scores for sugar (or sucrose) and honey are very similar.

### Better to go artificial?

Artificial sweeteners have a low GI score and therefore minimal effect on blood-glucose levels, but what concerns me is that "artificial" usually means "made from chemicals" and does not indicate any health benefits. Natural sweeteners may also have little effect on glucose levels, but they perpetuate the habit of eating sweet foods. If you can wean yourself off them, it is a much better option, and following the 10 Food Doctor principles should minimize any sugar cravings.

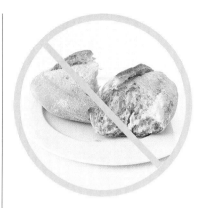

# Simple carbohydrates

Imagine eating a piece of mixed grain bread—by this I mean one with visible whole grains. You have to chew it, mix it with your saliva, and swallow it, allowing it to combine with the hydrochloric acid in your stomach. It passes into the digestive tract and the process of glucose extraction begins, along with the breakdown of vitamins and minerals. Since this type of bread is a complex carbohydrate, it scores around 50 on the glycemic index (*see pp.14, 47*).

If you had eaten white bread, which scores around 78 on the GI scale, the extraction of glucose would not have been slowed by the presence of whole grains. White-flour products have been over-processed until they lose their fiber—the fiber so essential for slowing down glucose extraction.

### What to avoid

You should minimize your intake of simple carbohydrates and avoid them when possible. So, reduce your intake of all sugars, many bread and flour products, white rice, white pasta, cereals, pastry, chocolate, alcohol, and sugary drinks. Alcohol is a simple carbohydrate and not only causes the usual changes to blood-glucose levels, but it can also distort your judgment in making food choices. Try to limit your alcohol intake and drink alcohol only with your meals.

Breakfast cereals break down very quickly. The typical dieter's low-calorie breakfast usually contains cereal, a glass of orange juice (after all, juice is healthy, isn't it?), and a cup of coffee (no milk, since you are watching your weight). This gives you two simple carbohydrates and caffeine, all in your first meal of the day. No wonder you feel tired and hungry again by mid-morning.

### Juiced fruit and vegetables

On the subject of juices, one of the key values of fruits and vegetables lies in their fiber content. Health officials worldwide recommend that everyone eat at least five servings of fruits and vegetables every day, yet juice counts as just one serving. Even if you drink 10 glasses of juice a day, they still count as one serving. This is because, although a glass of juice contains vitamins and minerals, it has no fiber. Yet fiber is just as important in combating disease as the antioxidants in fresh produce. In terms of the Food Doctor plan, the fiber is essential because it wraps around other foods and slows down the speed at which glucose is extracted. Whole foods, including fruits and vegetables, have far more intrinsic value than their derivatives.

Fruit juice, since it has no fiber to slow its conversion into glucose, has a high GI score, while whole fruit has a much lower score. If you like juice, just make sure that you eat some whole fruit alongside your juice to slow down the speed at which it is turned into glucose.

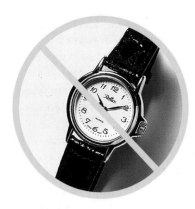

# Stress

I can't imagine a life without stress. In fact, it is probably an impossibility. Even the most laid-back person is certain to experience some stress, however minimal. As I sit at my desk, working to meet deadlines, my stress levels are elevated, although I may be unaware of this. The chemical changes can be occuring in my body without my noticing them.

## The role of glycogen

The stress response is simple. When the body senses that stress or danger is present, it releases a hormone called adrenaline from the adrenal glands (*see box, p.20*). Adrenaline affects your blood-glucose levels, triggering the production of insulin that effectively encourages your body to lay down fat. Stress can therefore result in weight gain. Since adrenaline inhibits digestion, it also prevents you from receiving all the nutrients you should from the foods you eat.

Stress has yet another way of affecting your weight. Adrenaline has the added effect of forcing stored glucose, known as glycogen, to be released from its stores in the muscles and liver. These glycogen stores are designed to provide quickly accessible short-term energy when needed during a stressful situation. The glycogen stores convert rapidly back into glucose and are released into the bloodstream to provide immediate energy to the muscles and brain which allows them to cope with the perceived stress or danger.

However, this glucose is not always needed, because common day-to-day stresses don't usually require us to flee or fight. This means that this surplus of glucose can then be stored, through a chain of biochemical changes, as fat.

## Recognizing stress

Stress or danger can take many forms. It is not necessarily the sort of executive or workplace stress that many of us associate with the word. In truth, anything you personally find stressful will trigger the stress response: from being late for school, running behind on an important work project, worrying about a family situation, money issues, or even weight problems. They all elicit the same response.

I am not suggesting that stress is something you can avoid, but try to remember that it is one of the elements and influences that force glucose levels to rise, which in turn triggers insulin production. It may help explain why you may have gained weight recently.

If you are suffering from stress, I advise you to pay even more attention to how you are dealing with the other triggers, such as caffeine and refined sugar, because you may find that you will need to eliminate these completely to compensate for life's unavoidable stressful situations.

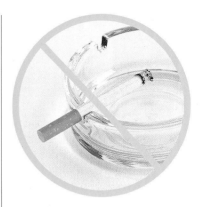

# Smoking

Cigarettes contain nicotine, a mild stimulant that triggers the release of adrenaline (*see box, p.20*), which impacts strongly on blood-glucose levels. I find that many smokers have problems managing their blood-glucose levels, but keeping them in check is, of course, an integral part of the Food Doctor plan.

## A poor start

Typically, a smoker may have their first cigarette at breakfast time, so blood-glucose levels spike right at the start of the day. I have also found that the majority of smokers skip breakfast because they have a cup of coffee and a cigarette instead. But breakfast sets the scene for the day. A small meal made from the right proportions of protein and complex carbohydrates effectively supplies fuel to encourage the metabolism to kick in for the day. Having a coffee and a cigarette instead will kill any feelings of needing food, so you eat less and your metabolism goes into "famine mode."

## Smoking and appetite

Most people are aware of the health risks associated with smoking, but I wonder how many people who smoke fully understand the link between smoking and excess weight. Traditionally, smoking is seen as an appetite suppressant, and surely that makes it a good thing for dieters? It is not that simple, I'm afraid. Aside from the link with rising and falling levels in blood-glucose, there is the problem that smoking reduces and sometimes completely removes the desire to eat. Then, when you quit smoking (which hopefully one day you will), your appetite returns and you find yourself eating much more than your metabolism is used to (*see pp.24–27*). The good news is that keeping glucose levels in check through regular eating, as advocated in the Food Doctor plan, can significantly reduce the level at which smokers need to replace nicotine with food when they finally quit.

At the risk of preaching, I ask my clients who come in for private consultations if they intend to smoke for the rest of their lives. Invariably, their answer is no. So then I ask when they expect the rest of their lives to begin. This is trite, I know, but it does help them to focus their minds on why they continue to smoke.

### How this diet helps

If you are a committed smoker, I suggest you keep a record by writing down the times of day you normally have a cigarette. Then try eating a little food frequently during the day, especially at those times when you usually have a cigarette break, still bearing in mind my recommended ratios of complex carbohydrates and protein. You may well find that your dependence on nicotine diminishes naturally, and this makes quitting the habit altogether a far easier task than you might have imagined.

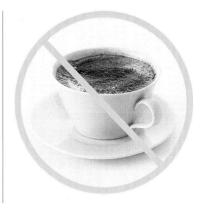

# Caffeine

Caffeine is found most commonly in drinks such as coffee and soda. To a slightly lesser degree, it is also present in tea and chocolate. Energy drinks are, of course, further significant sources.

These days, coffee-drinking seems to have become an integral feature of daily life: We're often grabbing a cappuccino or latte en route to work, or meeting a friend for a midmorning coffee at one of the many coffee shops that have sprung up in our towns.

Coffee (and caffeine) has become a social phenomenon, and drinking coffee repeatedly during the day has become the norm. But how does this seemingly innocuous beverage affect our weight?

### Highs and lows

Caffeine stimulates the production of adrenaline (*see box, p.20*) and can be addictive because of the "highs" and "lows" that follow. When adrenaline levels are elevated, we feel awake and able to work and function well. However, this feeling is always followed by a slump once the effect of the adrenaline wears off. This leaves us feeling sluggish and weary because we are no

longer able to sustain that high. The rise in blood-glucose levels, inevitably followed by a fall, leaves the coffee-drinker in that familiar position of feeling hungry or in need of more caffeine to try to recreate the high. Either way, no one, no matter how focused and strong-willed, is likely to make great food choices in this situation, because they feel tired and in need of a boost. Can you imagine craving some green vegetables and hummus midmorning after a breakfast of cereal and coffee? It's fairly improbable, isn't it? You are far more likely to crave a cookie or three, plus another cup of coffee.

### Curb the coffee

Coffee is readily available and popping out for a latte is more than socially acceptable—it is practically expected. I rarely drink coffee as I am aware of its negative effects, but I do recognize that its social associations have rendered excessive coffee-drinking apparently innocuous. Coffee is still a stimulant, however, and you must start thinking of it in that way. If you want to lose weight easily, consistently, and for the long-term, then reducing your intake of caffeine has to be part of the whole life-changing process. If you really feel you can't cut out the caffeine completely, limit yourself to one cup of coffee a day.

Keeping glucose levels in check by eating less food more frequently, and eating protein together with complex carbohydrates at every meal, including snacks, will minimize cravings and curb any desire for stimulants—including caffeine.

# Your metabolism

People so often blame their metabolism for their failure to lose weight, and it's true that the metabolism is a key factor in successful weight control. Understanding the impact of repeated dieting on your metabolism will help you avoid the pitfalls in the future.

I deal with clients who have a wide range of issues, but when it comes to those who seek advice solely for weight loss I will always ask them which diets they have tried. The usual response is "all of them." Of course they will have lost weight on all the diets they did but, needless to say, once they stop the restrictive way of eating prescribed by whichever diet they're trying and return to their normal eating habits, they gain back all the weight they lost and more. Sound familiar? This sort of dieting history can usually be traced back to being a teenager or young adult, and the most difficult part is helping clients understand that The Food Doctor plan is not actually a diet. I tell them this is the end of their "dieting" days, and I draw diagrams such as the insulin rollercoaster (*see pp.16–17*) and the six steps to a confused metabolism flowchart (*see pp.26–27*), and explain why the approaches they have tried so far have been unsuccessful in keeping their weight down in the long term.

When I first started incorporating this information into weight-loss consultations I found that people reacted quite strongly. The most usual response was one of familiarity and sometimes frustration at having been "on" diets for so long. There have been tears, nods of understanding, or smiles as the story seems too close to home. Let me explain why that is, and how repeated dieting might have led you to this point in your life.

## Your metabolic "set point"

We all have a "set point." This is the point at which your food intake creates exactly the same amount of glucose (*see p.26*) as your body requires for its day-to-day functioning. For example, let's assume that your set point is 2000 calories: The daily energy your body needs to walk, talk, digest, breathe, and think is 2000 calories, which is equal to the amount your body produces from the food you consume in an average

day. I don't usually like to think or refer to food in terms of its caloric value but it is useful in this context for ease of reference.

## How dieting affects your set point

Now, what happens to your set point when you alter that balance? As outlined below and illustrated in the chart on pages 26–27, dieting doesn't have the impact you'd like on your metabolism.

If we assume, for instance, that over time you have exceeded your energy requirements and have stored some fat, so you decide to go "on a diet" and cut down your calorie intake. You know that exercise burns calories, so you join a gym, take up running, start walking to work, or get off the bus a couple of stops earlier than you need to, to burn off more calories than you're eating.

So now your body has to release some of its stored glucose to meet the new exercise demand and compensate for your decision to decrease your calories. Once the glycogen runs out, fat stores are mobilized to turn the food that was stored away back into energy. So you lose a bit of weight in the first week or so although, as any long-term dieter will probably know, glycogen is stored in water so the weight you lose early on is the water that the glycogen was held in. But there's a bigger problem brewing. Your metabolism doesn't realize you are living in the 21st century. It thinks you are caveman or cavewoman. So it assumes that you are hitting a period of famine and compensates by going into "famine mode" (*see pp.26–27*), slowing itself down a little and lowering its set point to meet the new level of food intake.

Now you will find that your weight loss slows or even stops, which is pretty frustrating because a few days beforehand you'd been convinced that the diet

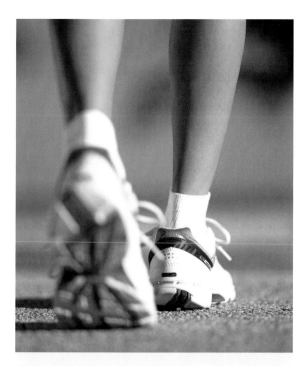

## THE BENEFITS OF EXERCISE

- Enhances metabolic rate and helps you burn body fat.

- Increases blood flow and helps improve cardiovascular function.

- Helps overall glucose management and tolerance, which reduces the need for insulin

- Reduces blood pressure.

- Encourages endorophin creation, which relieves anxiety and improves mood.

was working and worth sticking to. It is at this point that you are tempted to "break" the diet or "cheat," since you feel a little let down. Let's assume, however, that you are being strong-willed, and you decide to cut down a little more, and exercise more, too. Your weight loss speeds up again, but sadly, the set point lowers further as your food intake has dropped yet again. So now that your set point has lowered, your body has adjusted to a very restricted level of food intake that you need to stick to just to stay at exactly the same weight. This is not sustainable, enjoyable, or flexible and, worse

still, is unlikely to provide you with much energy. At this point you will start to get hungry, and so begins the cycle of self-blame and guilt for being hungry, or for not being able to control yourself (*see p.30*). For long-term dieters this tale is sadly familiar, but the lesson applies to everyone, long-term dieters and new ones alike—lose weight slowly at a sustainable rate if you want to be successful and avoid disrupting your metabolism.

### But what about the Seven-day Diet?

So, if dieting messes up the set point, why did I devise the Seven-day Diet in my previous book, *The Food Doctor Diet*? What is so different about it? Well, I included it as a "starter diet" for several reasons. The primary reason was to promote digestive health, and to introduce you to the 10 principles (*see pp.12–13*) in a structured way that showed you how easy it can be to follow them.

The Seven-day Diet is lower in calories than my Plan for Life (in the previous book) and the Daily Diet here. While it is a structured diet, you can be flexible about it if you prefer. There is no magic to it, just plain good sense and an ideal balance, so, should you prefer to eat the food for day 6 on day 3, or swap lunch for dinner on a specific day, or generally change meals around to suit your preferences, it doesn't matter: The most important elements stay the same.

So why is it different from other diets and why won't it mess up your set point? Simply because it still follows the 10 principles, it still guarantees sustained energy release throughout the day, and it's designed to last for a limited period only. The Seven-day Diet is not just about reducing calories, it's about eating the right foods little and often. You're never starving or short of fuel, so your body never retreats into famine mode. Ideally you should be aiming to follow the 10 principles in the long term, with the Seven-day Diet as a "kick-start" or "booster" option. I recommend that you do not follow the Seven-day Diet for longer than a week at a time, and do not repeat the Seven-day Diet more than once every six weeks. By doing this you will avoid upsetting your set point and not risk encouraging your metabolism to store an increased level of your food as fat.

### How exercise affects your set point

Often, just as people set themselves unachievable goals with diets that are unsustainable, they also try to maintain exercise routines that are equally unrealistic.

Gyms actually rely on the vast majority of their members *not* to come and, aside from every January, they usually get it right. Taking out a gym membership at the start of the year is just like starting a new diet, and often the two happen together. But by February, when your resolve has weakened as real life gets in the way, your food intake will revert to a previous pattern, and you won't be able to keep up the gym visits either. So another situation occurs in which you're setting yourself up to feel as though you've "failed" (*see p.30*).

It is absolutely true that we should exercise to enhance weight loss, but it helps to understand what happens in terms of metabolism when it comes to exercising. If we remind ourselves that food becomes glucose, which circulates in the blood and enters cells to be used as fuel

to create energy, then we can see that the more energy we require, the more glucose we will utilize. So surely the more we exercise, or the harder we do it, the more fat we will burn? No, not quite. All too often clients come to me specifically to lose weight and complaining that, aside from eating very little, they have also been exercising frantically each day. I hear tales of hour-long cardiovascular workouts, or 45 minutes sweating it out on treadmills or in aerobic classes, yet without the weight loss that you might expect from such exertion. And how many of you have been confused at the gym to find that one of the *lower* rather than higher settings on the machines is the one for "fat-burning"? I could never understand why it took a lower output of energy to burn fat—surely the faster you went the more weight you would lose?

## SIX STEPS TO A CONFUSED METABOLISM

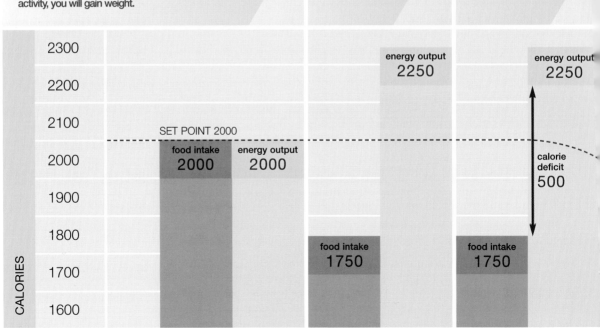

We all have a "set point"— a point at which your food intake is equal to your body's requirements for healthy day-to-day functioning. If your caloric intake is high, however, more food will be digested, and depending on how long you do this and your level of activity, you will gain weight.

**Your first diet**
So, for example, you have a metabolic set point of 2000 calories, but you're feeling a little plump so you decide to lose a bit of weight ...

**Cut calories**
To do this, you go on a quick crash-diet, lowering your intake to 1750 calories and increasing your exercise levels to 2250 calories ...

**Quick fix**
In a fair world, you'd lose weight due to the 500-calorie difference in food intake and energy burned—and for a week or two you do, as your set point hasn't yet adjusted to the reduced calorie intake and stays at 2000. But life isn't that fair ...

Unfortunately, it seems that, just as your set point can adapt to reduced food intake, so it may equally well be able to adapt to high levels of exercise. Your metabolism adjusts so that your body can sustain these levels without burning any extra calories. Therefore just as under-eating can have an effect on your set point, so can over-exercising.

## How to achieve a stable set point

Rather than frenetic over-exercising, it is actually sustained medium-level output (the "slow burn" that is important for enhancing your set point and encouraging the gentle and sustained release of fat, allowing it to be turned back into glucose so that your body can use it for energy.

The best way to do an exercise program is to find an achievable balance, an exercise you enjoy and a regimen you can follow even when you are short of time. This may mean joining a gym, getting together with a few friends to exercise, or just walking for a certain amount of time each day. The vital factor is to find something that you can slot into your life with ease and enjoyment. Don't allow exercise to become a huge hurdle to losing weight.

There is only one way to lose weight sensibly and slowly, which is to eat less food more frequently, combining complex carbohydrates and protein, as recommended in The Food Doctor plan, and to exercise at a steady level. This will ensure that your set point is maintained and avoid triggering your body's famine response.

**Set point adjusts**
After a few weeks, your restricted food intake of only 1750 calories triggers a "potential famine" alert in your body, which adjusts to function on that level by lowering its calorie needs. You are eating only 1750 calories a day, but your body has adjusted to fulfill all your energy demands on only that amount of calories ...

**After the diet**
You struggle to maintain a limited food intake of only 1750 calories a day, so you finish your diet and go back up to your "normal" intake of 2000 calories ...

**Famine mode**
BUT, as your set point is now only 1750, your body has a surplus of 250 calories. This is compounded by the fact that, as your body is in famine mode, it efficiently maximizes this excess into a glucose surplus. As energy output is only 1750, this surplus is stored as FAT ...

**The end result ...**
When you were dieting, your metabolism was alerted to possible famine and reset itself. Off the diet and in a time of relative abundance, it will store more of the food you eat as fat rather than make energy with it, in preparation for the next famine. The end result is that you gain back the weight you lost, and more.

To repair the damage long-term dieting causes your set point and adjust it back upward, you need a regular, steady supply of fuel combined with medium-level, sustained exercise. How quickly your set point recovers depends on many factors, such as the length and frequency of your diets, together with you caffeine intake and stress levels.

food intake
**2000**

food intake
**2000**

calorie surplus
**250**

SET POINT LOWERS TO 1750

food intake
**1750**

energy output
**1750**

energy output
**1750**

energy output
**1750**

# Think differently
## Portion proportion

For long-term dieters, or even for those who may be starting their very first diet, one issue that comes up frequently is that of just how much food they should be eating. Many people are worried about over-eating, and I can understand their concern.

I find that all too often long-term dieters cannot trust themselves not to overeat, which is why they can be so attracted to diets that cut out almost entire food groups. With such diets they feel that, even if they do over-eat, they are still "safe" as long as they stick to the permitted food groups.

Over-eating is linked to a feeling of guilt and failure. Traditional diets that restrict your food intake reinforce the whole scenario of "right" and "wrong," "good" and "bad"—a scenario that makes them unsustainable and inevitably doomed to failure (*see pp.30–31*).

### The ideal combination

When you understand the 10 simple principles of The Food Doctor plan (*see pp.12–13*) and, most importantly, eat frequently and combine the food groups in the ideal ratios, there is little danger of over-eating. The combination of ratios and timing will

## HOW IT ALL ADDS UP

| | BREAKFAST | MID-MORNING |
|---|---|---|
| **AVERAGE DIETER** | 25% | +0% |

**AVERAGE DIETER**

Many people follow what seems to be a healthy diet and, on the face of it, their food intake looks fine. There's nothing wrong with the foods, it's just the timing and the ratios that are wrong, resulting in blood-glucose lows, insulin production, and hunger.

25%

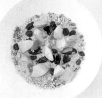

muesli with dried fruit, nuts, and chopped pear

+0%

mid-morning hunger

**FOOD DOCTOR DIETER**

Fuelling up frequently doesn't involve eating more than the average dieter, just spreading out the food intake and eating the right foods at the right time to maintain the body's energy supply and avoid the insulin rollercoaster (*see pp.16–17*).

20%

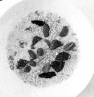

muesli with dried fruit and nuts (fewer nuts than above)

+10%

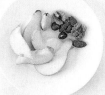

chopped pear with the remaining nuts from breakfast

automatically ensure that your meals and snacks will be large enough to satisfy you and supply the correct amount of glucose to get you through to the next meal (*see pp.18–19*). By adopting the 10 principles, you can avoid over-eating since you are not compensating for having been "bad" by skipping breakfast, for instance, or making up for the fact that you know you are planning to over-eat that evening.

## Eat frequently

For many dieters the idea of eating five times a day might seem a little alarming, because they are so used to limiting their food intake and feeling hungry. However, following the Food Doctor plan doesn't necessarily involve eating more food, it just

means spreading it out more evenly through the day (*see chart, below*). This ensures that blood-glucose levels stay even, energy is steadily released, and the body isn't pushed over the insulin threshold (*see pp.18–19*).

## Use your hands

You're probably familiar with those tedious diets that tell you exactly how many segments of grapefruit or slices of cucumber you can eat, regardless of your size, build or gender. The Food Doctor plan makes it so much easier. Instead of counting out each bit of food, you use your hands as a guide to portion size (*see box, right*). For each meal, I give the portion sizes of each food group as a percentage of your hand's surface area (*see for example p.46*).

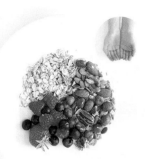

## A HANDS-ON APPROACH

Using hands as a portion guide works for us all, large or small, since hands are generally in proportion to bodies. For each meal I suggest simple portion sizes based on hand size.

| LUNCH | MID-AFTERNOON | DINNER |
| --- | --- | --- |
| +35% | +0% | +40%    =100% |

mid-afternoon hunger

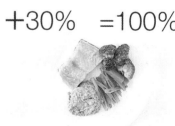

salad of red pepper, goat cheese, avocado, salad greens, and pine nuts

salmon with pea spread, steamed vegetables, and new potatoes

+30%    +10%    +30%    =100%

as above, but with potatoes: save some goat cheese and red pepper

rice cracker with the reserved goat cheese and red pepper

as above, but without the new potatoes, which you had for lunch

# Are you a "good" dieter?

Today, far too many of us think—consciously or subconsciously—that being slim is the sign of a good person. Conversely, being overweight is a sign that we are bad, or greedy, or out of control. We apply this judgement to such an extent that the word "fat" is an insult.

We can use the word fat to sabotage ourselves, implying that, being fat, we are also bad or greedy.

### The power of words
This attitude leads to the kind of dieting that invites the use of words and phrases like "good" and "bad," "cheat," "fall off the wagon," "start again on Monday"—I am sure you know them all. I cannot emphasize enough the value of taking a long, hard look at the words and phrases you use to describe yourself, and the way you talk about your dieting. You may well find that you are reinforcing a negative view of yourself and a distorted view of food and what it does for you.

Think how easy it is to make yourself feel bad when it comes to dieting and food choices. For example, you say things to yourself like "I should eat an apple mid-morning—after all, I am on a diet, but I want something else really." But, as you are on a diet, you deny yourself. A few minutes later you might think "I'll have raisins, after all, that's fruit so it's healthy." A few minutes later still you might think "I'll get the yogurt-covered raisins—

after all, yogurt is good for you, isn't it?" But in truth your choice is sugar masquerading as a snack. So you "ruin" your diet and, after a process of denial and indulgence, the "guilt" sets in and you think that you have ruined the whole diet for today anyway, so you may as well just eat "normally" and start "dieting" again tomorrow.

If you follow The Food Doctor plan, and eat at the right times in the ideal proportion, however, then you can get off the diet treadmill—and leave behind the language that goes with it—once and for all.

### Another layer of guilt
Exercise is another area in which we can set ourselves up to fail. Often, when people start a new diet, they galvanize themselves into action at the gym too. So alongside unrealistic and unsustainable diet, people try to maintain exercise routines that are equally unrealistic. But soon the real world gets in the way and the demands of work and family makes inroads into your exercise time, just as it does on the time you set aside for food preparation. When this happens, you revert back to your old

eating patterns and forego the gym visits. So another situation arises in which you're setting yourself up to feel as though you've "failed."

### The 80:20 rule
One of my 10 principles that people never have trouble remembering is the 80:20 rule—the principle that, as long as you follow The Food Doctor plan for 80 per cent of the time, you can "stray" for 20 percent of the time. This principle allows for the Real World, and it acknowledges that there may be times when you *really* want chocolate, for instance. That doesn't mean you're a "failure" or that you've "ruined" your diet: It's done, so just pick up and carry on with The Food Doctor plan at your next meal. Since the plan isn't a "diet," you don't "fall off" it: It's an eating plan for life, and it's always there in the background to help you make good food choices.

### On the right lines
Many of us try hard to be "good" and to stay on track. We've picked up various words of wisdom during the course of our dieting years and we feel "good" if we follow them. Sadly, many of these are myths (*see opposite*) and will only sabotage your attempts at weight loss—setting yourself up for more frustration and possibly even comfort-eating if your dieting cycle is particularly vicious.

Unless you feel the same **longing for broccoli**, the magnesium-craving theory isn't a viable **excuse for chocolate**

## "I eat lots of fruit"

Fresh fruit is an excellent source of fiber, liquid, minerals, and vitamins, including essential antioxidants. However, bear in mind that it is also rich in fructose, which is a type of sugar, albeit one with a relatively low GI value. Keep fruit intake under control, especially soft fruit, and ensure that there is no shortfall in nutrient intake by making sure you eat plenty of fresh vegetables.

## "I never eat eggs"

The high cholesterol content of eggs scares many people, but eggs are a complete protein food and, when poached, scrambled, or boiled, they make an excellent companion for complex carbohydrates. The fat in eggs is low in saturates so it counts as "good" fat. All in all, eggs fit well within The Food Doctor plan and are especially versatile.

## "I only have cravings for chocolate when I have PMS"

There is a theory that women crave foods rich in magnesium, e.g. chocolate, to help ease PMS. However, green vegetables also contain magnesium so, unless you feel equally desperate for broccoli, the magnesium-craving theory does not seem to hold. Sugar cravings can be minimized by following the 10 principles.

## "I only have salad for lunch"

Not all salads are created equal, and a traditional dieter's lunch-time salad, usually some lettuce, tomatoes, and cucumber, simply doesn't provide enough food intake. It is a very low-calorie meal that lacks any protein. As we know, however, you need higher levels of fuel to maintain your metabolic rate and avoid lowering your set point (see pp.24–27).

## "I love fruit juice"

Many dieters think that fruit juice will help them lose weight. If you squeeze your own juice, you will be familiar with the fibrous mess that you throw away. That fiber is as important as the juice and losing it is not part of my plan. If you do drink juice, always have it *in addition to* your regular fiber intake (that is, vegetables and whole grains). Do not replace meals with smoothies or juices—this will not help weight loss at all.

## "I've inherited a sweet tooth from my parents"

Some people do, of course, prefer sweet to salty foods, but inheriting a sweet tooth is unlikely. It is more likely that your sweet tooth is due to habit and upbringing rather than genes. Following the 10 principles which keeps blood-glucose levels even, which makes you less likely to want to indulge your sweet tooth.

## "I only drink black, sugar-free coffee"

Holding back on the sugar may seem virtuous, but there's another problem with coffee—its caffeine content. Caffeine is the dieter's enemy: It encourages glucose levels to rise, which affects your metabolic rate as well as triggering insulin production. This, as we know, will, in turn, encourage fat storage (see p.23).

## "I always choose red wine"

Most red wines are relatively rich in the nutrients that benefit the heart, so they're a "good" choice for dieters. However, alcohol has a high GI score and converts into glucose quite rapidly, so drink wine only with your meals, not before them! One or two glasses three times a week is enjoyable and acceptable on The Food Doctor plan (see p.145).

## "Spreads are healthier than butter"

In most diets butter is a villain and spreads are king. But some spreads are better than others —how do you know which are "good"? While many are fine, some are very artificial. I prefer the real thing—regular butter every time, in moderation (of course) and preferably unsalted. It is tasty, and will not overly upset The Food Doctor plan.

# Don't count calories

Are you one of those people who judges all food—without even realizing you do it—by its caloric value? If you regard food as calories and make your decisions about what to eat based solely on calorie content, then your food choices may not be healthy ones.

The calorie-counting method of eating fails to take into account the true value of food. While I am not unaware of the calorie content of food, I do feel that the value of food lies in more than just the number of calories it contains. In my clinic I have worked with a number of clients who can recount the calorie content of any food from memory. All their choices about what to eat are based on this, but in my opinion that gives rise to two serious issues—their relationship with food and their criteria for judging its value (see also pp.42–43).

### An unhealthy relationship

Firstly, food can end up becoming an obsession. What should I eat today? Have I had too many calories? Should I be saving some for later? If this is you, then ask yourself if this approach has actually served you up to now. Are you the weight you want to be, or do you still battle? Do you slide off the wagon sometimes and indulge in ice-cream or pizza, and then feel guilty for not being able to control yourself? If so, where does that leave you? In my experience, it makes you feel as if you have failed, and nothing is more likely to send you back to making poor food choices than feeling bad about yourself (see pp.30–31).

Then there is the problem of the reduced-calorie foods available. Take a look at the list of ingredients in a typical ready-made low-calorie meal and you will see elements that you wouldn't add if you were making the same meal at home, such as modified starch, salt, and preservatives. Low-calorie meals tend to be processed and sugared—the opposite of what I feel smart eating is all about.

### The true value of food

Calories are one way of measuring what you are eating, but if you make food choices based solely on whether a food will make you fatter or thinner, then, to be blunt, you have missed the point. The foods that will enhance your health and digestion and keep the body functioning at optimum levels are not necessarily those that are low in calories. This doesn't mean you should ignore their calorie values, but rather make it just one of the ways in which you choose what to eat instead of it being the first and most important factor.

Here's an example. If you're focusing purely on calories, you might choose low-calorie cereal with skim milk, black coffee, and juice. However, these are all notoriously low in fiber and protein and rich in simple carbohydrates, which means they convert from food into glucose rapidly. This provides only short-term energy, it is highly likely that you'll be hungry again by mid-morning. The rest of the morning is then spent trying not to eat, or berating yourself for being hungry ("What's wrong with me?" "Why can't I control myself, it's only a couple of hours until lunch?"). If you had ignored the calorie count and eaten a breakfast that included fiber and protein instead, such as muesli with nuts and seeds, or even peanut butter on toast, the foods would have broken down into glucose more slowly and provided energy longer to avoid both the hunger and also the common mid-morning dilemma—whether or not you can eat again soon.

My advice is: Put calories to the back of your mind and choose your food based on a way of eating that will serve you better in the long run. In time, it will become second nature (just as counting calories did). Foods can then be judged in terms of taste, consistency, and—most importantly—nutritional value. Let food work for you, not the other way around.

**Healthy food** is not necessarily **low-calorie food**, yet that is how many of us define the **value** of **what we eat**

# Calories versus nutrients

If you've been counting calories for some time, you probably haven't eaten an avocado in ages, since it is high in calories. But that ignores its nutritional value. A low-calorie dieter might favor the diet drink with zero calories, but with zero nutrition too (*see below*).

Dieters who count calories can fall into the trap of viewing food merely as the sum of its caloric value, with nutritional value ignored. This leads to poor food choices. For example, oily fish that is full of essential fats and vitamins would be ignored in favor of "spending" the calories on food with fewer nutrients in it.

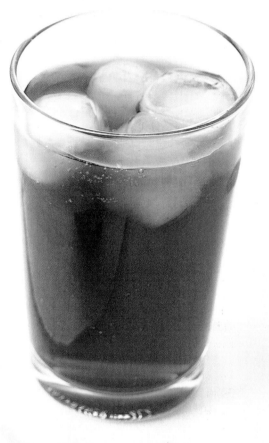

### Diet drink
The diet drink may have no calories, but it is also "empty" of any value in terms of nutritional benefits. It is also likely to be packed with chemicals and caffeine.

energy 0.4kcal
protein 0g
fiber 0g

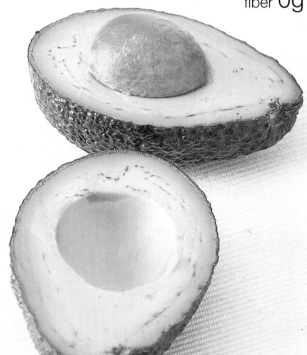

### Avocado
The calories in an avocado come from its mono-unsaturated fats, which are important for healthy body function. An avocado also contains other nutrients such as potassium and vitamins A, E, and B[6], making it full of "nutritional" calories.

energy 340kcal
protein 4.8g
fiber 16.2g

# Feeling the pressure

One of the difficulties of following a weight-loss program is keeping to it while facing the pressures (and pleasures) of everyday life: families to feed at home, for instance, or work commitments, or socializing with friends.

Losing weight is an emotional issue, both for you and for those people around you, many of whom are likely to have strong opinions about what you are doing. I have heard many accounts from clients of their friends or family being cynical of yet another diet or, worse still, being full of advice about how they "should" be eating. The latter reaction usually stems from people who believe that, if something worked for them (or their friend/ mother/cousin), then it should work for you and you should be following their diet instead of what you have chosen to do for yourself.

### Have faith in yourself

It is imperative that you manage peer pressure. Friends and relatives must understand that your dieting days are over, and that your new way of eating is one that takes into account overall good health, together with sustainable weight loss.

People around you may try to tempt you with foods that you are generally avoiding, with comments or excuses such as "You deserve it" or "I made it especially for you" or even "You have lost weight, you're

allowed a treat." You need to be aware that these comments will not help, and you must learn to become immune to them.

The Food Doctor plan is designed to become second nature, to be so easy and familiar that before long you will make food choices almost automatically that are appropriate for weight control and overall good health. You can do this alone, with friends, family, or in groups. If you feel that you need more support, then visit www.thefooddoctortips.

### Fitting in the family

The principles of The Food Doctor plan (see pp.12–13) can be adopted for the whole family. The food is not diet food, so you don't have to subject your family to eating low-calorie or unappetizing food. If you prepare food, following my ideal proportions of complex carbohydrates and protein, and eat at the recommended times, then you can feed the family in the same way as you feed yourself.

My eating plan will encourage consistent concentration and energy levels, so it is ideal for children too. I do not suggest that children follow the Seven-day Diet (from my earlier

book, *The Food Doctor Diet*), but they can eat according to the 10 principles of The Food Doctor plan, although for those under 16 I suggest 25–30 percent protein per portion, rather than the 40 percent recommended for adults.

While we are talking about the children, don't let your family be an excuse to "fail" your diet. Say, for example, your children fail to finish a meal, as is their wont, so you end up finishing it and the guilt sets in —again (see pp.30–31). If you ensure that their meal combines protein with complex carbohydrates, then you can happily pick at some or save it for one of your snacks. This may seem obvious, but it works and, as long as you are not eating too late in the day, or have already had your snack, then it is entirely appropriate within The Food Doctor plan.

### The last resort

You will have already come across the 80:20 rule (see pp.12–13). This principle is designed to enable you to continue following The Food Doctor plan after any odd "blip," without the guilt or negative emotions associated with most diets.

And none of the usual excuses work either. Opposite are some of the many phrases you'll have heard or used as a dieter in the past, along with solutions to help you avoid those obstacles in the future.

The **Food Doctor** plan is designed to become **second nature** so that you automatically make **good food choices**

## "I made it especially for you"

Hmm. Tricky, whether it's your partner who's been slaving lovingly in the kitchen, or your mother, or your own child. If you can "adapt" what's being offer to fit the 10 principles, do so: If not, simply follow the 80:20 rule and return to The Food Doctor plan for your next meal. And try dropping gentle hints so it doesn't happen again...

## "You've done really well on your diet, you deserve a treat"

Sometimes friends or family can try to be encouraging while actually sabotaging your diet. But you're not on a "diet," this is an eating plan for life and nothing is banned, so don't worry too much. If you can, however, try to ensure that "treats" are related to a form of indulgence other than food.

## "But you're on vacation..."

So what? Different countries may have different dishes, but they are all made of the same food groups, so you should still find it easy to stick to The Food Doctor plan on vacation. Also, once you're used to following the 10 principles, you will find that there is no sense of deprivation or restriction about your food, so a "break" from your eating plan is unnecessary.

## "I don't have time to cook differently for the family"

Unless you are on the Seven-day Diet, which is not recommended for children, there is little reason to cook differently for your family. All of the recipes in the Daily Diet are suitable for children, so serve them up without a second thought. Just give those under 16 a slightly smaller percentage of protein (25–30 percent).

## "But my family won't eat what I eat!"

Your family need not know that they're eating diet food. Look at the various recipes and menu suggestions in this book: Would your family guess that they were being given "diet food" if you served these up? As you know, The Food Doctor plan is not a diet, it's a healthy eating plan without an end date, so simply follow the 10 principles when preparing their meals and yours.

## "But my partner likes eating out"

Who doesn't? Eating out doesn't need to be a minefield for dieters. In the Daily Diet there are plenty of strategies to help you enjoy a restaurant meal according to the 10 principles (*see pp.144–47*). If worse comes to worst, there's always the 80:20 rule. The important point is that you return to eating healthily after your evening out.

## "I don't have time to shop and cook properly"

With a little preparation, you can easily avoid time issues. The Daily Diet recipes are very simple and many take less than 20 minutes to make. There are also many time-saving strategies, such as planning ahead, organizing your shopping, making meals in minutes, and cooking in batches (*see pp.36–37*).

## "It's easier just to skip a few meals"

You may think that simply skipping a few meals, particularly breakfast and lunch, when you might be eating alone anyway, is the easiest way to lose a few pounds. Sadly, any weight you lose this way will only be short-term, since this is not a sustainable way of fueling your body, and you're just storing up problems (*see pp.24–27*).

## "Eating out a lot is part of my job"

The Food Doctor plan can easily accommodate this situation. Usually I can find something on most menus that fits the food group profile, and I can exercise portion control by using my hands as a guide (*see pp.28–29*). Don't be afraid to ask the waiter to alter a dish slightly, and resort to the 80:20 rule if you have to (*see also pp.144–47*).

# Time is no excuse

As you will know by now, many of the readily available convenience and snack foods you can buy do not fit in with The Food Doctor plan. There are various ways of making your own easy meals to make in minutes, however, that fulfill all the requirements of the Daily Diet.

One of the main reasons people find it difficult to follow any diet is lack of time—which is why they buy convenience foods in the first place.But pre-prepared food is rarely healthy because of the potentially high levels of fats, salt, or sugar. With The Food Doctor plan just a little effort is required when it comes to food preparation.

### Plan ahead

This is simpler than you think. The more familiar you become with The Food Doctor principles (*see pp.12–13*), the more you will see how easy it is to adapt. The secret is to have the right foods available: You will need a well-stocked pantry and an eye for any ready-prepared foods that are suitable for the Daily Diet. Planning ahead is easy with the shopping list I have prepared for you (*see pp.44–45*), and inspiration for quick and easy menu ideas and options can be found throughout this book.

You can be as untraditional as you want in your food choices, as long as the ratio between protein and complex carbohydrates is correct (*see pp.46, 60, 70, 73*).

### Simple short-cuts

If you are too busy during the day to make lunch, or lack the time or energy to cook properly when you are at home in the evening, instead of resorting to pasta, try experimenting with leftovers (*see opposite*), or turn to your freezer or pantry for a quick meal. In this book there are many recipes that you can make in only minutes using ingredients from the pantry if you have had no time to shop (*see pp.134–43*).

A freezer is a helpful tool for the busy dieter. Foods such as shrimp, peas, baby corn cobs, lima beans, green beans, and fish all freeze well and can be called upon for a quick stir-fry when shopping and cooking time is limited (*see pp.108–09 for recipe suggestions*).

Many of my recipes, such as the ratatouille (*see p.96*) and the soups, can be prepared in batches and frozen into individual portions of home-made "convenience foods." The sauce recipes also fit this strategy well (*see pp.94–95, 143*). In fact, add a small can of beans to the tomato sauce, heat, and serve on whole-wheat toast for a traditionally English "quick dish" of beans on toast!

Ready-made store-bought soups are another good option when you are short on time, but check for hidden "extras" in the ingredients. Buy a vegetable- rather than cream-based soup, add some extras yourself in the form of protein, such as fish chunks, chick-peas, sliced chicken or shrimp, and you have a filling, almost instant Daily Diet meal.

As long as you wash them well, ready-prepared salad greens are an acceptable time-saver, especially if you have a jar of home-made dressing (*see pp.114–15*) in the fridge. Buy some plain, cooked chicken to go with it and you have convenient, no-cook meal with minimal effort, in minimal time, that still fits the plan.

If a club sandwich is your only option for lunch, choose one made from whole-wheat or rye bread, with a protein filling such as turkey or tuna, then remove the a layer of bread from each half and enjoy the sandwich while reducing your intake of carbs. If you have a baguette, remove the top layer of bread to create an open sandwich (*see pp.82–83*). This will ensure the best ratio of healthy protein filling to less healthy carbohydrate bread layer.

So, with a little advance planning —making sure you have the right foods in your fridge, freezer, and pantry—preparing Daily Diet meals and snacks can actually be quick. Lack of time is no excuse.

Take time to **plan ahead** and many of **The Food Doctor's** meals and snacks can be almost **"instant"**

# Use leftovers to save time

The recipes in this book, or those from the original *Food Doctor Diet*, can nearly all be eaten cold the next day. Leftovers make instant healthy snacks, or they can be turned into delicious new main courses.

## Chicken and meat leftovers

Cut chicken and other meats into small cubes or fine strips, then combine them with fresh vegetables, such as cubes of cucumber or tomato, or chopped sun-dried tomatoes and olives, if you are resorting to the pantry. Add some herbs and toss in one of my dressings (*see pp.114–15*). Use as follows:

- as a healthy topping for crackers
- as an interesting protein dish tossed with some salad greens and chopped raw vegetables
- to add essential protein to your lunchtime pasta or couscous

## Fish leftovers

Place the cold fish in the blender, add 2–3 tablespoons live natural yogurt, a teaspoon of olive or walnut oil and some fresh dill. Blend briefly to make a thick paste. Take care not to over-blend, or it will become too thin. Try other herbs and vary the consistency to suit your own taste. I recommend experimenting with other herbs, peppercorns, juniper berries, or saffron. Use as follows:

- as a topping on crackers for snacks
- on whole-wheat toast for lunch
- as a filling for a small lunch-time baked potato
- to make a delicious dip for crudités
- as a stuffing for tomato, avocado, or sweet pepper
- wrapped with salad greens in a buckwheat pancake (*see p.104*)

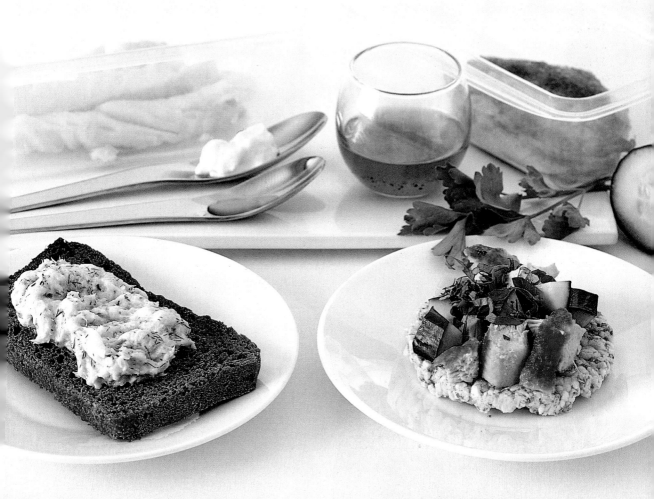

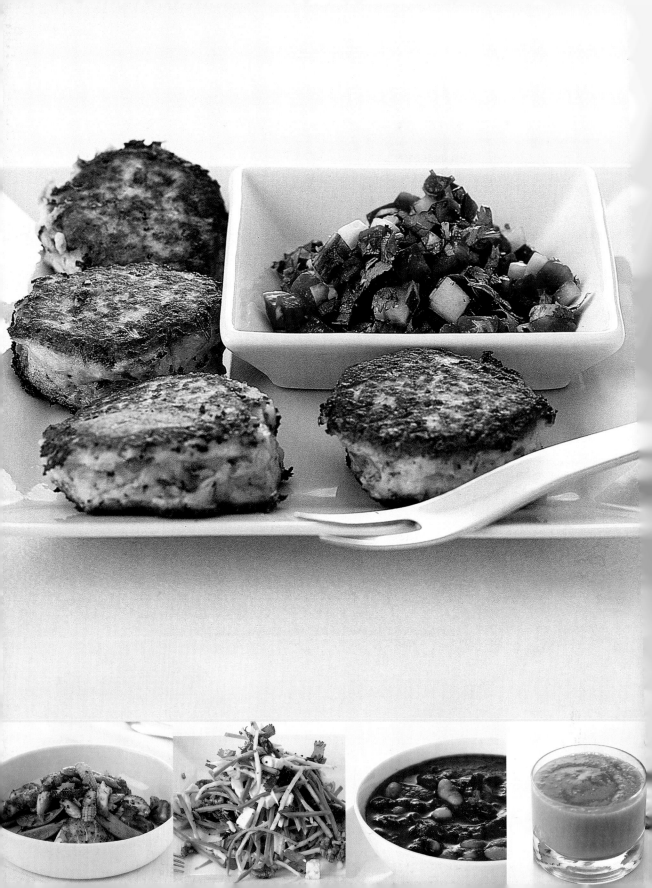

# Everyday eating

Here you will find all the essential tools you need to make smart food choices in every given situation—at work, at home, in a hurry, out with friends—and for every meal—breakfast, lunch, dinner, or a snack. With more than 100 recipes to choose from and many more ideas and variations to browse through, this part of the book shows you how easy it is to follow The Daily Diet.

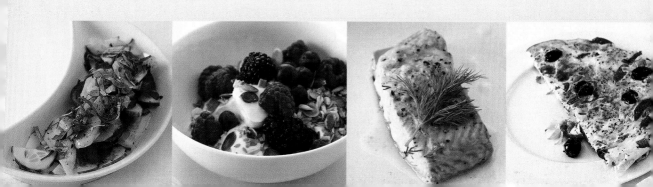

# Buying healthy food

There are so many confusing labels out there and so much ingenious packaging designed to make you feel good about what you're buying. But will it actually help you to control your weight and maintain it? Here's my guide to the shopping maze.

There's no doubt about it: Preparing your own food from scratch is the safest way to ensure that there are no "hidden extras" in your meals. But, in the real world, we are often short of time and desperate for convenient options, particularly if they offer a promise of weight loss too. That's when we fall prey to the pitfalls of shopping and make poor choices in our food selections.

### Always read the label
When you first start with The Food Doctor plan try to take a little extra time to shop, looking at the foods you usually buy. Check labels for their carbohydrate, fat, sugar, modified starch, and high salt content. Avoid the many forms of sugar that are innocently hidden behind names such as sorbitol, malt extract, or corn syrup. There are more than 16 ways to describe sugar (*see*

## Lack of **time** to shop or cook **doesn't have** to mean lack of **good food**

*p.20*), and it's the same story for fats. The trick is to look for the healthy, essential fats derived from sources such as seeds, nuts, plants, and oily fish, and to avoid the saturated fats and trans fats (often listed as hydrogenated or partially hydrogenated vegetable oils).

The food industry aims to make its products appealing, so terms such as "reduced fat", "low-fat" and "lite" are used to tempt you to buy anything from ready-made meals to a simple container of yogurt. In reality, many of these claims are not regulated by law. Nor do these products necessarily contain fewer calories or "healthier" ingredients: In many cases, where the fat comes out, sugar goes in to give the product flavor and substance.

Since one of my 10 principles (*see pp.12–13*) is to avoid sugar, foods labeled as "no added sugar" might seem tempting. Again, however, beware, as this simply means that sugar has not been added as an extra ingredient: It does not mean there is no sugar present in the product.

### The food industry
So how have things come to this? Why all the tricks and misleading labeling? The blame lies equally with the food industry and with ourselves. I know that food manufacturers come in for a lot of criticism, and I feel that it's generally with good reason. Like any business, however, they have a right to make a profit and to run their business in a manner that reduces their costs and maximizes their profit. They are often public companies and therefore have an obligation to their shareholders to be successful. The food manufacturers make foods that are saleable, and so they make them as rich in flavor as they can (which can mean added salt, sugar, or other additives), and use ingredients that are consistently available and have "added value." This means that, for example, while a simple potato is worth a few pennies, if you chop it finely, deep fry it in oil, add some salt, and package it in an appealing way, that same potato is now worth many times more than the original. Throw in some celebrity advertising and suddenly the potato is a potential pot of gold.

The same can be said for the ears of corn that become a breakfast cereal, nuts that get honey-coated and roasted, simple meal recipes that become high-value frozen dinners (with instructions to "pierce film several times to ensure product is hot before serving") or fruit that is juiced, mixed with yogurt, and turned into a smoothie. Due to the high profit margin, the food manufacturers can afford heavy advertising, often with celebrity endorsement, that suggests that their product and their product alone will help you lose weight, or is a great alternative to a cooked breakfast for those of us who are short on time, or whatever.

In this way, the food industry has to a large extent influenced what we all weigh. OK, so they may have taken a few liberties with exact truths over the years, allowing us to think that the phrase "low-fat" on a package will result in our bodies becoming low in fat, or suggesting that a carbonated, caffeinated, artificially sweetened drink deserves the word "diet" in its name, but all they really gave us was what we wanted. And what we wanted was food that was going to keep us healthy, full, satisfied, and thin, yet could be prepared in seconds with little effort or thought on our part. No easy task.

Our own role in the food industry cannot be under-estimated. We have contradictory attitudes. As well as expecting food to be cheap and available to us all year round, we want it to be good for us. Yet we will pay more for fatty, sugared, and salted added-value foods, because we are too busy to cook. Food scares outrage us, yet our high expectations of the food industry makes it almost inevitable that quality may suffer from time to time.

## A question of time

The time factor is of great relevance when it comes to weight loss. I realize we are all busy, and that life today brings endless pressures, but when people consult me about weight loss, it often turns out that they have been using convenience foods as staple foods. Low-fat snacks and ready-made meals allow them time for other things and, with so much else to do in life besides worrying about food, it's easy to see how tempting it can be to believe the labels and try the shortcuts. But resorting to processed foods is not going to provide the answers: Only sensible eating can do that.

I firmly believe that, if we can learn the principles of good eating, then we can start to enjoy food properly. By putting food higher up on the list of priorities, and by apportioning time to cook and prepare it, we can make better choices affecting our weight and overall health. It doesn't have to be disruptive (many of the recipes in this book can be made in only 10 minutes or so). It simply means making sure that you have a healthy attitude toward food, you are organized in your shopping, and you keep the 10 principles in mind when you prepare meals. Lack of time doesn't have to mean lack of good food (*see also pp.36–37*).

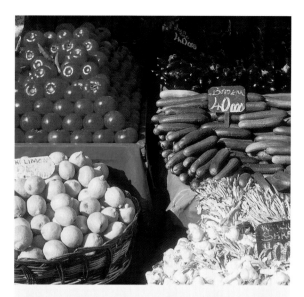

## HELP YOURSELF

Willpower and motivation are all well and good, but the act of food shopping can cause even the most determined of us to waver. Make shopping easier on yourself with the following tips:

- We've all heard the one about not shopping when you're hungry, and it's a good rule. If you can avoid shopping when you're already hungry you'll find it much easier to make good food choices.

- If you know the layout of your supermarket, you know which aisles are full of cookies and chips, don't let yourself go down those aisles. This way, no cookies will mysteriously end up in your shopping basket.

- Try to make a list of what you need before you go shopping and stick to the items on it (*see pp.44–45 for the "perfect" shopping list*), but don't be blind to interesting new foods. You could aim to add one new food a week to your shopping basket—just be sure to make healthy choices.

- If time allows, don't let food-shopping become a dull, routine chore. Shopping at places such as farmer's markets, greengrocers, butchers, etc,will help you avoid the lure of the racks crammed with sugary, fatty foods and frozen dinners.

# Compare and contrast

There are so many different diets to try, but how well do they work and what are the health costs? In our eagerness to find a simple weight solution, many of us embrace diets that are, in fact, unhealthy.

There is a wide range of diets on the market, many of which can be very hard to follow and impossible to stick to. Many focus on calorie-counting or excluding food groups. So if someone tells you of a different diet that allows you those forbidden food foods, then of course it's tempting—all those foods that have been off your list could be on it again. The problem is that you are still on a diet, with its own list of forbidden foods. So inevitably, after a while, you will start to crave the foods that your new diet does not allow.

Ultimately I feel that any traditional "diet" is doomed to fail, since by its nature it has a beginning, middle, and end, and is something you try as an *alternative* to your usual eating patterns rather than as an *improvement* on them. The Food Doctor plan, in contrast, includes all food groups. I'd like you to avoid sugar, but even that isn't forbidden, thanks to the 80:20 rule (*see pp.12–13*). The balance between the food groups means that no foods are off-limits, so cravings will be minimal.

The problem with low-calorie and high-protein diets is that they distort your concept of the value of food, so that you rate foods merely by their caloric value or carbohydrate content. Thus, for instance, the essential fats that your body needs for optimum health and weight loss are labeled as "fattening" and avoided by low-calorie dieters, who prefer to "spend" their calories on eating more food with a lower value. Faced with a choice between a few nuts or a few low-calorie cookies, they choose the latter and forget that the nuts supply essential fats, promoting weight loss, healthy hair, skin, and nails, while the cookies are loaded with sugar. They may be "low-fat" but they have a very high GI score (*see p.14*). A comparison of two other diets with the Food Doctor plan clearly shows its benefits (*see right*).

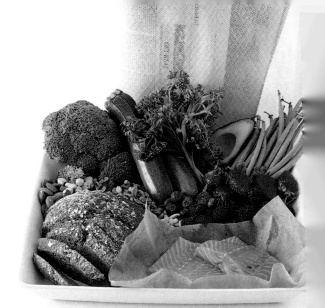

## The Food Doctor plan

### PROMISE

An eating plan for life, with no deprivation, hunger pangs, or calorie-counting. No food group is excluded, and there is a healthy balance of fiber, protein, and complex carbohydrates to ensure optimum health.

### OUTCOME

- Since no food group is excluded, the plan provides balanced nutrition for optimum health.

- Eating regular meals promotes a stable metabolism and avoids hunger, with its inherent dangers to willpower and food choices.

- Intake of fruit and vegetables is high, ensuring plenty of fiber and antioxidant consumption.

- Its practical, realistic eating pattern means that you're unlikely to "cheat" or find it too hard to do, and it's a plan for life, so you don't have to stop.

- You are encouraged to eat "healthy" fats such as the essential fats derived from fish, nuts, and seeds.

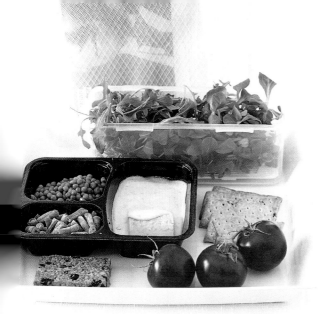

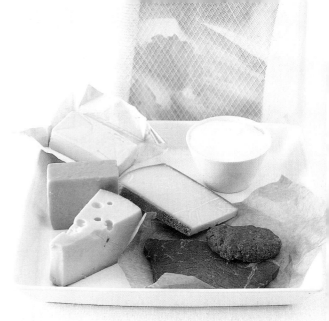

# Low-calorie diet

### PROMISE

A low-calorie diet based upon the caloric values of foods and upon the idea that, if you eat fewer calories than you use, you will burn your body fat as energy and thus lose weight. But the human body is far too complicated to respond to calorie-counting. You can end up on a form of starvation diet yet still fail to lose any weight.

### OUTCOME

- Food becomes merely the sum of it's caloric value, with nutritional value ignored (*see pp.32–33*), leading to poor food choices and increased risk of health problems.

- Even essential fats that are vital for optimum health and weight reduction are labeled as "fattening" and avoided.

- Restricted food intake slows down your metabolism (*see pp.26–27*), making it hard to sustain any initial weight loss.

- When you return to eating "normally," your metabolism will still be in "famine mode" and so you gain more weight than you originally lost.

# High-protein diet

### PROMISE

A high-protein diets designed to limit your intake of carbohydrates. They usually have an "induction phase" of all-fat-and-protein intake, with carbohydrates to be introduced later in the program. During this initial phase, weight loss is most noticeable. In practice, many people stay in this induction phase (*see p.18*) because of the successful short-term weight loss.

### OUTCOME

- Restricted carbohydrate consumption means that you are unlikely to achieve the recommended five portions of fruit and vegetables per day in your dietary intake.

- Long-term use of the induction phase means intake of fiber may be poor, leading to constipation which may increase your risk of colon cancer.

- Poor intake of antioxidants due to lack of fruit and vegetables increases risk of diseases such as cancer, heart disease, and arthritis.

- Increased danger of high intake of saturated fats, which may lead to high cholesterol and thus heighten the risk of heart disease.

# The ultimate shopping list

Keep the following foods, or the majority of them, stocked in your kitchen and you will easily be able to prepare a healthy Food Doctor meal.

## Grains & wheat

- [ ] Brown rice
- [ ] Buckwheat flour
- [ ] Buckwheat noodles
- [ ] Couscous
- [ ] Gluten-free flour
- [ ] Millet flakes
- [ ] Oats, jumbo
- [ ] Quinoa
- [ ] Rye/whole-wheat bread

## Beans

- [ ] Canellini beans, canned
- [ ] Chickpeas, canned
- [ ] Flageolet beans, canned
- [ ] Lentils, French, green, red, canned or dried
- [ ] Lima beans, canned
- [ ] Mixed beans, canned
- [ ] Mung beans, dried
- [ ] Red kidney beans, canned
- [ ] Split yellow lentils, dried
- [ ] Split yellow peas, dried

## Nuts & seeds

- [ ] Cashews
- [ ] Hazelnuts
- [ ] Pine nuts
- [ ] Pumpkin seeds
- [ ] Sesame seeds
- [ ] Sunflower seeds
- [ ] Walnuts

## Herbs

- [ ] Basil
- [ ] Bay leaves
- [ ] Chives
- [ ] Cilantro
- [ ] Dill
- [ ] Fennel
- [ ] Lemon grass
- [ ] Marjoram
- [ ] Mint
- [ ] Mixed herbs, dried
- [ ] Oregano, dried
- [ ] Parsley
- [ ] Rosemary
- [ ] Sage
- [ ] Thyme

## Spices

- [ ] Black pepper
- [ ] Caraway seeds
- [ ] Cardamom pods
- [ ] Cayenne
- [ ] Chili powder
- [ ] Cinnamon, ground
- [ ] Cinnamon, sticks
- [ ] Cloves
- [ ] Coriander seeds
- [ ] Cumin seeds
- [ ] Curry powder
- [ ] Fennel seeds
- [ ] Five-spice powder
- [ ] Ginger (fresh)
- [ ] Ginger powder
- [ ] Mustard seed (black)
- [ ] Nutmeg
- [ ] Onion powder
- [ ] Paprika
- [ ] Poppy seeds
- [ ] Star anise
- [ ] Turmeric

## Oils

- [ ] Avocado oil
- [ ] Olive oil
- [ ] Sesame oil
- [ ] Walnut oil

## Pantry essentials

- [ ] Anchovy paste
- [ ] Black olives
- [ ] Carrot juice
- [ ] Coconut, creamed
- [ ] Coconut milk
- [ ] Honey
- [ ] Horseradish sauce
- [ ] Mixed vegetable juice
- [ ] Mustard, Dijon
- [ ] Mustard, wholegrain
- [ ] Peppers in olive oil
- [ ] Ratatouille, canned
- [ ] Soy sauce
- [ ] Stock, fish
- [ ] Stock, vegetable
- [ ] Stock powder
- [ ] Sun-dried tomatoes in olive oil
- [ ] Tapenade, black
- [ ] Tapenade, green
- [ ] Thai fish sauce
- [ ] Tomato paste
- [ ] Tomatoes, canned
- [ ] Vinegar, balsamic
- [ ] Vinegar, cider
- [ ] Vinegar, white wine
- [ ] White wine
- [ ] Worcestershire sauce

## Fruit

- [ ] Apples
- [ ] Apricots
- [ ] Blackberries
- [ ] Blueberries
- [ ] Grapefruit
- [ ] Kiwis
- [ ] Lemons
- [ ] Limes
- [ ] Oranges
- [ ] Pears
- [ ] Raspberries

## Vegetables

- [ ] Arugula
- [ ] Avocados
- [ ] Bean sprouts
- [ ] Beets
- [ ] Broccoli
- [ ] Cabbage, green
- [ ] Cabbage, green, red and white
- [ ] Carrots
- [ ] Celeriac
- [ ] Celery
- [ ] Chinese cabbage
- [ ] Corn, baby
- [ ] Cucumbers
- [ ] Eggplant
- [ ] Fennel
- [ ] Garlic
- [ ] Green beans
- [ ] Leeks
- [ ] Lettuce, romaine or cos
- [ ] Mixed salad greens
- [ ] Mushrooms, white and brown
- [ ] Onions, yellow and red
- [ ] Parsnips
- [ ] Peas, frozen
- [ ] Peppers, red, yellow, and green
- [ ] Peppers, fresh chili
- [ ] Rutabega
- [ ] Scallions
- [ ] Shallots
- [ ] Snow peas
- [ ] Spinach
- [ ] Sprouted seeds
- [ ] Squash, butternut
- [ ] Sugar snap peas
- [ ] Sweet potatoes
- [ ] Tomatoes
- [ ] Tomatoes, cherry
- [ ] Watercress
- [ ] Zucchini

## Dairy

- [ ] Cream cheese, low-fat
- [ ] Eggs
- [ ] Feta cheese
- [ ] Goat cheese
- [ ] Manchego cheese
- [ ] Milk
- [ ] Parmesan cheese
- [ ] Plain yogurt
- [ ] Tofu, silken (both firm and soft)

## Meat & fish

- [ ] Anchovies, canned
- [ ] Chicken breasts
- [ ] Haddock
- [ ] Mackerel
- [ ] Prosciutto
- [ ] Salmon, fresh fillets
- [ ] Salmon, smoked
- [ ] Scallops
- [ ] Shrimp, cooked
- [ ] Squid
- [ ] Swordfish
- [ ] Tuna, canned
- [ ] Tuna, fresh
- [ ] Turkey
- [ ] White fish fillets (cod, haddock, etc.)

# The right proportions

You can be as creative as you want about what you eat for breakfast, as long as you stick to the Food Doctor rules about food groups and proportions.

Cup both hands together slightly so that both are showing about 80% of their total surface area. This should give you an indicator for how big your portions should be. Your breakfast should make up about 20% of your daily total food intake.

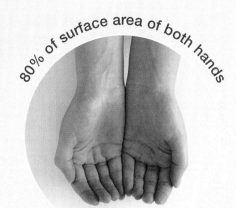

80% of surface area of both hands

## 30% complex starchy carbohydrates

such as rolled oats, sugar-free cereal, or wholegrain bread

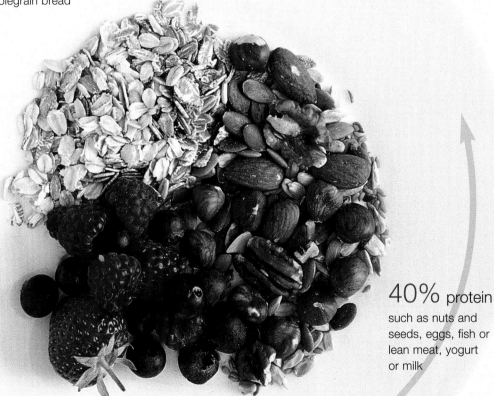

## 40% protein

such as nuts and seeds, eggs, fish or lean meat, yogurt or milk

## 30% complex carbohydrates

such as fruit

# Breakfast

The old saying that breakfast is the most important meal of the day couldn't be more true in terms of The Food Doctor plan. Skipping breakfast altogether or eating a high-carbohydrate breakfast is a sure-fire recipe for weight gain.

There is a very good reason why one of my 10 principles recommends not skipping this meal. By eating breakfast you can stimulate the ideal metabolic rate for the day, as long as you make smart food choices. Furthermore, skipping breakfast is likely to set the scene for subsequent highs and lows during the day (*see pp.16–17*).

## A bad breakfast

A typical breakfast of cereal, black coffee, and orange juice contains little fiber, and very little or not enough protein. Since each of these foods falls into one of the categories that encourages an increase in blood-glucose levels and thus triggers insulin production, having a combination of these foods leads to far swifter response, which in turn leaves you feeling hungry sooner than you need to. So, you have a bowl of cereal for breakfast, and are hungry again by the time you get to work or have finished getting the kids to school. Cereals and convenience breakfast foods, which now include branded cereal bars,

which have a pleasant aura of health about them, are sugary and refined, with inevitably high GI values (*see pp.14–15*). However convenient these foods may be, they will not help you lose weight in the long term, so you are going to have to look elsewhere and put a little more effort into this all important first meal of the day.

## A good breakfast

If you like to eat cereal, simply choose a sugar-free cereal, then add some fruit and protein— perhaps some nuts and seeds. Adding fiber in the form of fruit, and protein, in the form of nuts or seeds, while reducing the simple carbohydrate element, changes the meal into one that contains 40% protein and fits the portion breakdown (*see opposite*).

It really doesn't matter whether you want cereal or steak for breakfast, as long as you have the correct food groups in the right ratios. Match your portion size to your hand size, too, and you can start the day any way you like.

### IDEAL CHOICE GRAINS AND BREADS

The breads and grains below are those that have the lowest GI ratings.

| | | | |
|---|---|---|---|
| Whole-wheat pasta | 38 | Bulgur wheat | 45 |
| Rye bread | 40 | Sourdough rye | 48 |
| Pumpernickel | 41 | Brown rice | 50 |
| Oatmeal | 42 | Wholegrain bread | 51 |
| Toasted muesli | 43 | Multigrain cereal | 55 |

### POOR CHOICE GRAINS AND BREADS

Avoid refined options such as those below, as they are low in fibre and have high GI ratings.

| | | | |
|---|---|---|---|
| Corn flakes | 85 | Bagel | 72 |
| White bread | 78 | Crumpet | 69 |
| English muffin | 77 | Croissant | 67 |
| Cocoa puffs | 77 | White or regular pasta | 61 |
| Waffles | 76 | White rice | 60 |

# Menu ideas

# Quick breakfasts

Browse these ideas for inspiration on how to create a perfectly balanced, nutritious, and tasty breakfast. They are quick to make and perfect for a rushed weekday morning.

## Fruit smoothie

- **fruit** two handfuls of any fruit, such as strawberries, blackberries, raspberries, plums, apricots, peaches, nectarines, cherries, or mangoes

  and

- **yogurt** a couple tablespoons of plain, low-fat, or fat-free yogurt

  and

- **seeds** about a tablespoon of seeds, such as pumpkin, sunflower, or sesame

  and

- **low-fat milk** enough milk to create the right consistency

## Quick classic cereal

- **cereal** about 4 tablespoons of cereal, such as plain (unsweetened) corn flakes, bran flakes, or barley flakes

  and

- **nuts** a small handful of mixed nuts, such as Brazil nuts, pecans, hazelnuts, macadamias, and almonds

  and

- **low-fat milk** a little more than is needed to moisten the cereal: Choose from cows' milk or soy milk

## Nut butter on toast

- **toast** two slices of toast, such as as pumpernickel, wholegrain, or rye bread

  and

- **sugar-free nut butter** a thin coating of either cashew, peanut, or almond butter

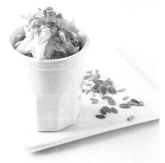

Yogurt with fruit and seeds

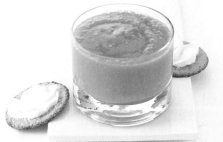

Fruit smoothie

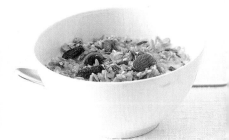

Quick classic cereal

## Cheese or ham with bread

- **bread**  2 slices of bread, such as rye, wholegrain, or pumpernickel

  and

- **cheese**  a few thin slices of any hard cheese, such as Parmesan, Manchego, or cheddar

  or

- **meat**  a few slices of lean meat, such as chicken, turkey, or ham (not honey-roasted or sugar-cured)

## Yogurt with seasonal fruit and seeds

- **yogurt**  a couple tablespoons of plain, low-fat, or fat-free yogurt

  and

- **fruits**  a handful of chopped fruit, such as apples or pears, or whole berries, such as cranberries, blackberries, raspberries, or blueberries

  and

- **nuts and seeds**  a tablespoon of any combination of nuts and seeds, such as almonds, walnuts, and sunflower, or pumpkin seeds

## Eggs with toast or crackers

- **eggs**  two eggs poached, scrambled, or soft-boiled

  and

- **toast or crackers**  a slice of toast (such as pumpernickel, wholegrain, or rye), a rice cake, or piece of crispbread

# Menu ideas

# Leisurely breakfasts

Sometimes, especially on the weekends, breakfast can be a more indulgent affair. These recipes are quick and not too involved, but are more of a treat than an everyday event.

## Sweet pancake

- **basic pancake wrap** one pancake wrap (*see p.104*)

  and

- **fruit** a handful of sliced fruit, such as pears, plums, apples, blueberries, nectarines, kiwi, papaya, and mangoes

  and

- **yogurt** a couple tablespoons of plain, low-fat, or fat-free yogurt

  and

- **nuts** a tablespoon of chopped nuts, such as almonds or pecans

## Fish-topped toast

- **fish** one serving of oily fish, such as salmon, sardines, mackerel, or tuna (in moderation), chopped or mashed very roughly

  and

- **tomato** one chopped tomato, or some chopped roasted sweet red or yellow peppers, mixed in with the fish

  and

- **toast** one slice of toast, such as pumpernickel, wholegrain, or rye bread

## Eggs with steamed spinach

- **eggs** two eggs, either poached, scrambled, or soft-boiled

  and

- **spinach** a generous handful of steamed spinach or other steamed or grilled vegetables, such as bok choi, kale, or asparagus

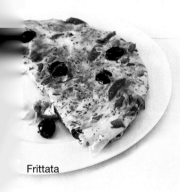

Frittata

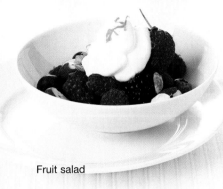

Fruit salad

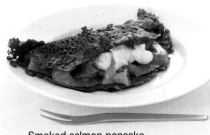

Smoked salmon pancake

## Fruit salad

- **fruit** a handful of fruit, such as blackberries, strawberries, blueberries, apples, apricots, red- and blackcurrants, peaches, and mangoes

and

- **yogurt** a couple tablespoons of plain, low-fat, or fat-free yogurt

or

- **nuts and seeds** a tablespoon of mixed chopped nuts and seeds, such as Brazil nuts, almonds, and sunflower seeds

## Frittata

- **frittata** choose from recipes such as leek, Mediterranean, mushroom and tomato, red pesto or sweet potato and dill (*see pp.58, 86 and 87*), or make your own recipe with ingredients you have available, such as olives, Manchego cheese and anchovies, or smoked mackerel, onion, and corn

and

- **toast** one slice of toast, such as pumpernickel, wholegrain, or rye bread, with a thin spread of butter if you wish

## Savory pancake

- **basic pancake wrap** one pancake wrap (*see p.104*)

and

- **egg and smoked salmon** one poached egg and a few pieces of smoked salmon

or

- **goat cheese** a handful of soft goat cheese with some arugula, or a chopped baked tomato

# A good breakfast ...

All the rumors you've heard about how essential this meal is are true: It really is important to start the day with a healthy breakfast.

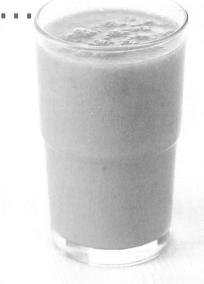

## The usual choice

**Peach and papaya smoothie** How can a drink made almost entirely from fruit be improved upon? Added extras, such as honey and fruit juice can send the GI score soaring. This smoothie is lacking protein so it is important to also make some additions.

**Strawberry yogurt with banana** Surely a yogurt and some fresh fruit is a healthy option? Well, yes, but only if you make the right choices and keep in mind the ratio of protein to complex carbohydrate. Yogurt alone won't provide enough protein, and you should check the label for sugars or other additives along with the flavoring. Don't forget, too, that some fruits are better than others at providing steady glucose conversion throughout the morning.

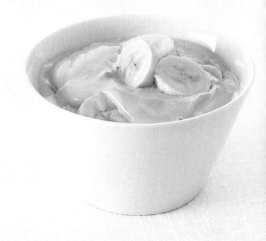

**Cereal and milk** A processed breakfast cereal with milk, even if you've chosen a high-fiber cereal, such as bran flakes, is not a good choice, since your protein quota is most definitely not being fulfilled, and the processed cereal will convert into glucose rapidly and produce only short-term energy. Many commercial cereals are laden with sugars, fats, and salt, too.

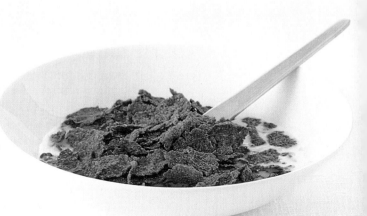

# ...can be even better

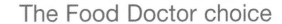

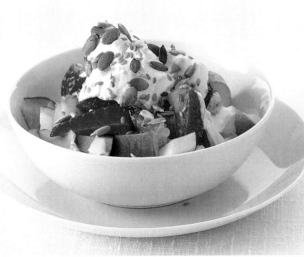

## The Food Doctor choice

Some fruits have higher GI ratings than others, and adding fruit juice raises them even further. Cut out the honey because it is pure sugar.

- Choose fruits with a low GI score, such as plums, apricots, strawberries, blackberries, and pears.

- In place of fruit juice, use full-fat milk to create the right consistency.

- Add some seeds and soft tofu to the blender to increase the protein content.

- See my smoothie recipe on page 57.

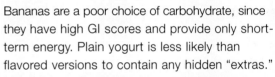

Bananas are a poor choice of carbohydrate, since they have high GI scores and provide only short-term energy. Plain yogurt is less likely than flavored versions to contain any hidden "extras."

- Choose fruit with a low GI score, such as apples, apricots, strawberries, and pears.

- Sprinkle some seeds and/or nuts on your yogurt to be sure that it meets the protein requirements and keeps you feeling full.

- Add your own flavorings, such as a pinch of cinnamon, with a mixture of fresh apple and hazelnuts, to add variety.

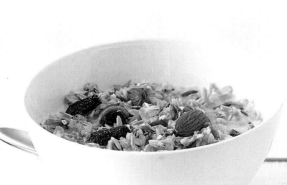

Switching to muesli will ensure that your breakfast is broken down into glucose relatively slowly, so you shouldn't feel hungry too quickly.

- Make sure your muesli is rich in nuts and seeds to bump up the protein quotient.

- Make sure that you don't have too much dried fruit and hidden sugars in any commercial muesli you buy.

- Why not make your own muesli? It can easily be stored for up to four weeks in an airtight container (see p.49).

# Crunchy yogurt

Here is a fresh take on breakfast muesli, based on fresh fruit rather than the dried ones in regular breakfast cereals. Serves two.

**ready in 10 minutes**

½ pint (300ml) plain yogurt

2 tablespoons rolled oats, toasted (*see note*)

¼ cup (60g) mixed seeds (choose from sesame, sunflower, poppy, or pumpkin)

2 tablespoons soft fruit, such as blueberries, raspberries, or blackberries

Divide the ingredients between two bowls, putting the yogurt in first and the soft fruit in last so that they are on top of the other ingredients.

Note: To toast oats, spread them thinly on a baking tray and put them on the top rack of an oven (preheated to 350°F/180°C/gas mark 4) for about 8 minutes until browned. It is a good idea to toast several portions of oats beforehand and store them in an airtight container for up to 2 weeks.

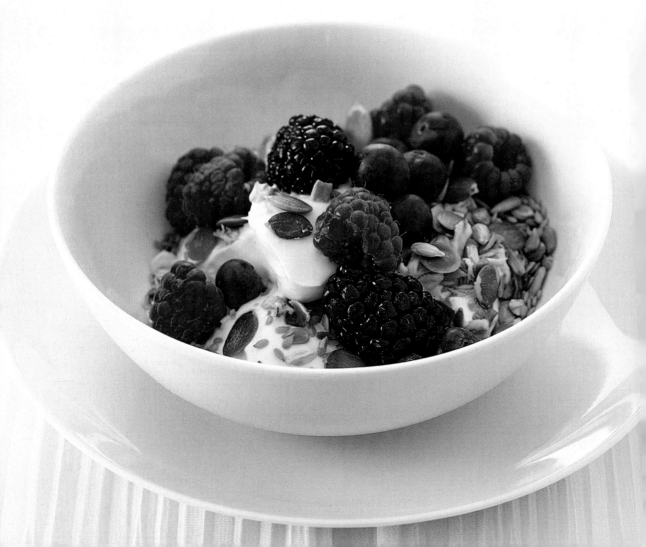

# Red and green scramble

You can make an extra portion of the egg mixture and use it cold as a spread on rice cakes or toast for a mid-morning snack. Serves two.

ready in **15** minutes

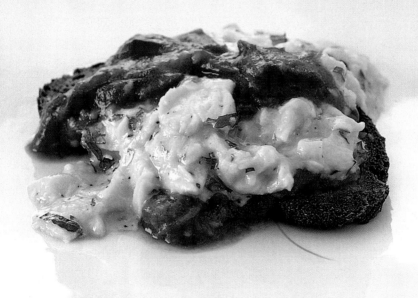

1 tablespoon olive oil

2 tomatoes, roughly chopped

4 eggs, lightly beaten

2 tablespoons chopped fresh parsley

Freshly ground black pepper, to taste

2 slices rye bread, toasted

Heat the oil in a nonstick skillet over medium heat. Add the tomatoes and cook for about 2 minutes until softened, then remove them and set them aside on a plate. Pour the eggs into the same pan and stir gently until soft curds form. Fold in the softened tomatoes, chopped parsley, and some black pepper. Serve over toast.

# Hot millet cereal

A pear would be just as good as an apple in this hearty breakfast cereal. Since millet can be tricky to find in some stores, alternative cereals that work equally well are suggested. Serves two.

ready in **15** minutes

¼ cup (75g) millet flakes (or barley flakes, buckwheat flakes)

½ pint (250ml) water

¼ cup (75g) plain yogurt

1 large crunchy apple, cored but not peeled, and sliced or grated

2 tablespoons pumpkin seeds

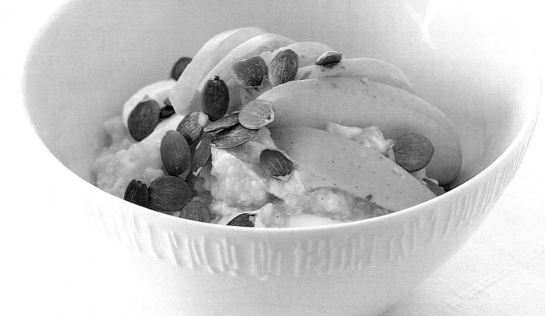

Place the millet flakes and water in a small saucepan, mix them together and bring them to a boil. Quickly reduce to a simmer and cook the mixture gently for 5–10 minutes, until all the water is absorbed and a soft porridge results.

Stir in the yogurt to make a creamy porridge.

Divide the porridge between two bowls and top each with the apple and the pumpkin seeds. Serve immediately.

# Sunshine smoothie and rice cakes

This smoothie is a wonderful color and not too sweet. It is also packed with beta-carotene. The ingredients make nearly 1¼ pints (about 700ml), enough to serve two at breakfast and have some left over for a midmorning snack.

ready in **10** minutes

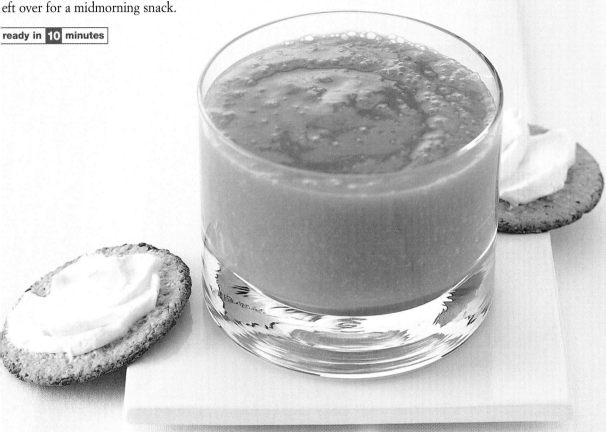

4 fresh apricots, halved and pitted

1 mango, halved and pitted, with flesh cut into chunks

Juice of 2 oranges (approx. 3½fl oz/100ml)

1 cup (250ml) carrot juice

2 tablespoons wheat germ

Put the apricots, mango chunks, juices, and wheat germ in a blender and blend until the mixture is smooth. Drink 7fl oz (200ml) for breakfast, with two rice cakes or crackers per person topped with low-fat cottage cheese or cream cheese to provide protein.

Note: The remainder of the smoothie can be used for a quick snack during the morning. If it is too thick, just blend it with 3½oz (100g) silken tofu and add some more carrot juice.

# Mushroom and tomato frittata

This slow-cooked omelet makes an excellent weekend breakfast dish. Teamed with a green salad, it also works well as a main meal. Serves two.

ready in **10** minutes

1 tablespoon olive oil

Approx. ¼ cup (60ml) brown mushrooms, sliced

4 eggs

2 tablespoons plain yogurt

Freshly ground black pepper, to taste

1–2 tablespoons chopped parsley

2 medium tomatoes, chopped

Heat the olive oil in a nonstick skillet, add the mushrooms, and soften over medium-low heat.

Break the eggs into a bowl, beat them lightly, and add the yogurt, black pepper, and chopped parsley. Mix everything together well. Stir in the chopped tomatoes.

Pour the mixture over the mushrooms in the skillet, making sure that the filling is evenly spread over the bottom of the pan. Cook over medium-low heat until the bottom of the frittata is firm. To cook the top you can either slide the whole pan under the broiler for a couple of minutes or slide the frittata onto a plate and invert back into the pan. Divide the frittata and serve with whole-wheat, multi-grain, or rye bread.

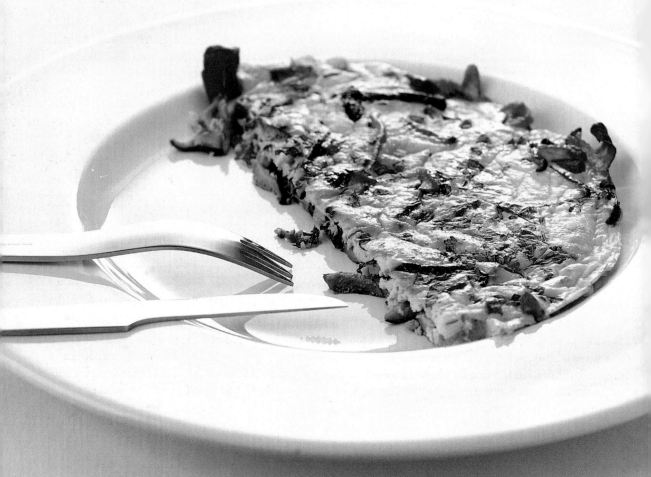

# Smoked salmon and poached egg pancake

**BREAKFAST**

These delicious egg and salmon wraps make good use of this book's basic pancake recipe. The wraps are ideal breakfast-time food, but also make great snacks or lunchtime treats. Serves two.

ready in **10** minutes

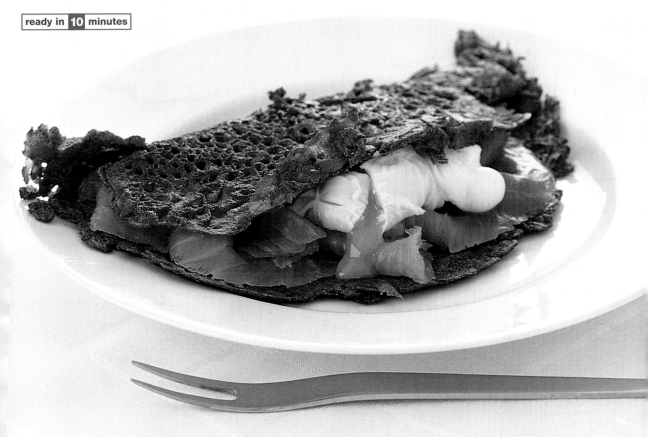

2 eggs

2 pancake wraps (*see p.104 for basic pancake wrap*)

2 slices smoked salmon (approx. 2oz/60g total weight)

Juice of ½ lemon

Fill a pan with water, add a dash of vinegar, and bring it to a simmer. Break each egg into a saucer and slide them into the simmering water. Poach the eggs until they are firmly set, but not hard. Remove the eggs with a slotted spoon and set aside.

Heat a small nonstick skillet and wipe or spray it with olive oil. If the pancakes are already cooked, heat them one at a time in the pan on both sides. If you are cooking the pancakes fresh, cook one side, then flip over.

While you are still cooking/heating the second side, place a slice of smoked salmon on one half of the pancake, squeeze the lemon juice over it, and slide an egg on top. Fold the pancake in half over the filling and repeat for the second pancake. Serve immediately.

# The right proportions

A snack simply needs to be a combination of protein and carbohydrates. It doesn't have to be complicated or time-consuming. It's up to you to be imaginative and find protein and carbohydrate combinations that you like.

Use one hand, slightly cupped, so that it's showing about 80% of its surface area, as an indicator for how big your portion size should be. Your midmorning and midafternoon snack should each make up about 10% of your daily total food intake.

80% of one hand surface area

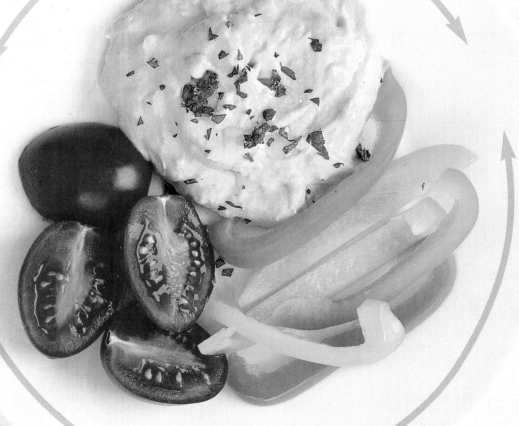

**40%** protein
such as the beans in this hummus, nuts and seeds, eggs, fish, or lean meat

**60%** complex carbohydrates
such as fruits or vegetables

# Snacks

The Food Doctor plan relies upon a number of principles, and eating less food more often is one of the most important of these. Fueling up frequently keeps the metabolism running smoothly and supplies you with a steady energy supply.

Many clients come from a "three square meals a day" background and are nervous about eating between meals. They worry that if they eat five times a day they will eat far too much—a concern that stems from a history of denial and excess. With The Food Doctor plan, however, the danger of overeating is reduced. since you will be eating exactly the same amount as you would with the traditional three meals a day, but dividing them into five smaller meals (see pp.28–29).

## Avoid the insulin rollercoaster

Eating mid-morning and mid-afternoon is vital to keep your energy levels constant and avoid the "lows" leading to cravings and poor food choices. When you're hungry, for example, rather than drink coffee, which will raise blood-glucose levels and suppress the normal hunger response, you could have a simple snack that will supply nutrients and slow-releasing energy instead. It doesn't have to be complicated, nor does it have to be traditional or hard work (see pp.62–65 for suggestions).

Snacks can be as simple as a cracker or two with unsweetened nut butter, or a piece of fibrous fruit, such as an apple or pear, with some nuts or mixed seeds. Eating a small handful of seeds with a piece of fruit will supply minerals, nutrients, essential fats, and protein, while the fruit offers fiber and yet more nutrients. Perhaps of more relevance to weight loss, the combination of protein, essential fats, and fiber is one that is broken down slowly by the body so you will limit hunger, and let blood-glucose levels rise gently to avoid triggering a surge of insulin.

Pre-made deli food makes an ideal base for good snacks, such as hummus with some celery or a carrot. It doesn't have to be beautiful, you don't need plates, the table doesn't need to be set—you just open a container of hummus and scoop some out with a vegetables. Leftovers also make great snacks (see pp.36–37). For example, if you have chicken and vegetables for a main meal, make a little more and save it for snack-time.

### IDEAL FRUIT CHOICES
These fruits make great snack choices because they have a low GI rating.

| | | | |
|---|---|---|---|
| Apricots | 20 | Peaches | 30 |
| Grapefruit | 20 | Strawberries | 32 |
| Cherries | 22 | Pears | 35 |
| Plums | 22 | Oranges | 35 |
| Apples | 30 | Figs (fresh) | 35 |

### POOR FRUIT CHOICES
Their quick conversion into sugar and high GI rating make these fruits poor choices.

| | | | |
|---|---|---|---|
| Watermelon | 72 | Raisins | 65 |
| Dried fruit | 70 | Figs (dried) | 61 |
| Pineapple | 66 | Black grapes | 59 |
| Cantaloupe | 65 | Kiwi | 58 |
| Bananas | 65 | Orange juice | 57 |

# Menu ideas

# Snacks to pack

Often the key is convenience, both in making the food and how handy it is to eat on-the-go. These snacks take minutes to prepare but stave off hunger for much longer.

## Fruit and nuts

- **fruit** a piece of fruit, such as an apple, pear, peach, or nectarine, or a couple of apricots, plums, clementines, or mandarin oranges, or a handful of grapes, or berries

and

- **nuts** five or six nuts, such as almonds, walnuts, hazelnuts, pecans, or Brazil nuts

## Hummus with crudités

- **hummus** a tablespoon of hummus, preferably home-made

and

- **vegetable crudités** a handful of raw chopped vegetables, such as carrots, red peppers, cucumber, cauliflower and broccoli florets, cherry tomatoes, scallions, or red, green, yellow, or orange peppers

## Spreads

- **spreads** a tablespoon of of spreads, such as sweet potato and goat cheese, mushroom, tapenade and tofu or lima bean and mustard (*see pp.66–67 for recipes*)

and

- **toast or crackers** a couple of thin slices of toast such as whole-wheat or rye bread, or two crackers, such as crispbreads, or rice cakes

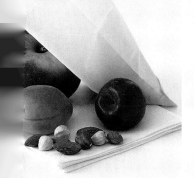

Fruit and nuts

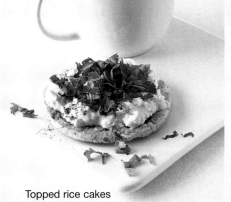

Topped rice cakes

Hummus with crudités

## Crackers spread with nut butter

- **crackers** two crackers, rice cakes, or a couple pieces of crispbread

  and

- **sugar-free nut butter** a thin coating of either cashew, peanut, or almond butter

## Yogurt and fruit

- **yogurt** a small container of natural low-fat or fat-free yogurt

  and

- **fruit** a handful of soft berries stirred into your yogurt, such as strawberries, raspberries, or blackberries, or some chopped fruit, such as apricot, mango, plum, papaya, nectarine, apple, or pear

  and

- **seeds** a sprinkling of seeds, such as sunflower, sesame, or pumpkin

## Topped rice cakes

- **dip or spread** a tablespoon of your choice of dip, preferably home-made (for a selection of dips such as fish, avocado, or pepper and sun-dried tomato, *see pp.68–69*)

  or

- **crackers** two crackers, rice cakes, or a couple pieces of crispbread

# Quick and easy snacks ...

Snacks keep the body going with a steady
energy supply. If you snack regularly, you'll be
less likely to overeat at mealtimes or make
poor food choices due to hunger.

## The usual choice

**Dried fruits and an "energy bar"** I can almost
sense your disappointment at being told this isn't
a perfect choice as it might seem very healthy.
There are still a few substitutions you could make,
however to turn this into a truly healthy snack.

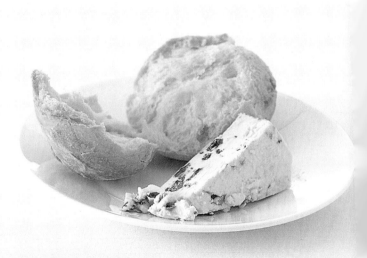

**Bread and cheese** Many of us find it hard
to resist a chunk of fresh bread with
cheese: With a few careful substitutions
The Food Doctor Daily Diet allows you to
continue enjoying such pleasures, while
still controlling your weight.

**Low-fat cookies** Surely dieters can eat
cookies if they are labeled "low-fat"?
Unfortunately not. To create flavor, low-
fat options are often packed full of sugar
and sweeteners, guaranteed to trigger
insulin production. However convenient
this option seems, there is always a
price to pay.

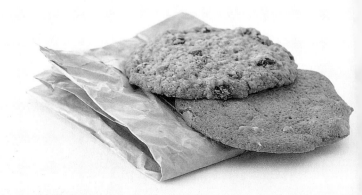

# and how to improve them

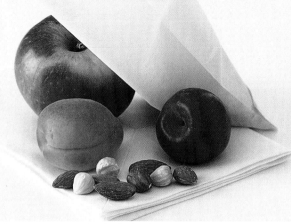

## The Food Doctor choice

Many energy bars are packed with sugars and cheap ingredients instead of the nuts and seeds required to supply protein. Dried fruits are a poor-choice of carbohydrate because they have a high GI rating.

- Choose fruits that have slower glucose conversion, such as apples, plums, or apricots.
- Instead of an energy bar, eat five or six hazelnuts or almonds with your piece of fruit.
- As a tasty alternative protein source, try a handful of mixed sunflower and pumpkin seeds.

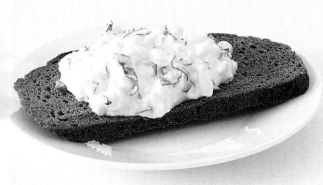

White bread is a poor choice since it is low in fiber and has a high GI value. Instead, try rye bread or oatcakes since this allows you to vary your grain intake.

- Goat cheese is lower in fat and makes a good substitute for cow's-milk cheeses.
- Avoid blue and aged cheeses because they contain mold that can lead to excess yeast.
- Low-fat cottage cheese, possibly flavored with some fresh herbs or scallions, makes a tangy alternative topping.

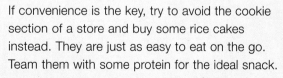

If convenience is the key, try to avoid the cookie section of a store and buy some rice cakes instead. They are just as easy to eat on the go. Team them with some protein for the ideal snack.

- The quickest accompaniment to your crackers is to layer some lean ham on top.
- Hummus is a great protein option. If you have time, make it yourself so it's additive-free.
- Chopped cucumber mixed with linseeds, mint and plain yogurt makes a healthy topping.

# Spreads

These spreads are as easy to make as they are filling and versatile. Spread on rice cakes, or on a piece of rye bread or melba toast, they make delicious wholesome snacks. A spoonful of your favorite spread can also spice up lunch or dinner—serve it on the side or as a topping.

## Pea, ginger, and tapenade spread

ready in **15** minutes

5oz (150g) frozen peas, thawed

½in (1cm) piece fresh ginger, peeled and finely grated

2 tablespoons olive oil

Juice of ½ orange

Grated zest of ½ orange

Grated zest of ½ lemon

2 scallions, finely chopped

1 garlic clove, finely chopped

2oz (60g) silken tofu

5 teaspoons green tapenade (*see p.148*)

Juice of ½ lemon

Freshly ground black pepper, to taste

Plain yogurt (optional)

1 tablespoon chopped fresh mint

Put the peas, ginger, olive oil, orange juice, zests, scallions, and garlic in a heavy-bottomed pan. Bring to a boil, reduce the heat, and simmer gently for about 10 minutes, until the peas are well cooked.

Pour the mixture into a blender, add the tofu, and blend to make a slightly rough spread. Alternatively, add the tofu to the pan and use a hand blender to mash it. Turn the spread into a bowl and stir in the tapenade, lemon juice, and black pepper to taste. If the spread seems too thick, stir in a little olive oil and/or some plain yogurt. Finally, stir in the mint.

## Sweet potato and goat cheese spread

ready in **30** minutes

1 cup sweet potato (approx. 7oz/200g), peeled, and coarsely chopped

1 tablespoon olive oil

2 garlic cloves in their skins, tips chopped off

2½oz (75g) soft goat cheese, crumbled

Lemon juice, to taste

Freshly ground black pepper, to taste

1–2 tablespoons finely chopped fresh cilantro

Preheat the oven to 180°F/350°C/ gas mark 4.

Put the chopped sweet potato in a baking dish with the olive oil and garlic cloves. Cover the dish and put it in the preheated oven. Bake for about 25 minutes, or until the sweet potato pieces are soft.

Squeeze the soft garlic cloves out o their skins and tip into a bowl with the sweet potato. Add the goat cheese and mash everything together until well blended, but no reduced to a smooth purée. Add lemon juice and pepper to taste and plenty of chopped cilantro.

Red lentil, cumin, and turmeric spread

Lima bean and mustard spread

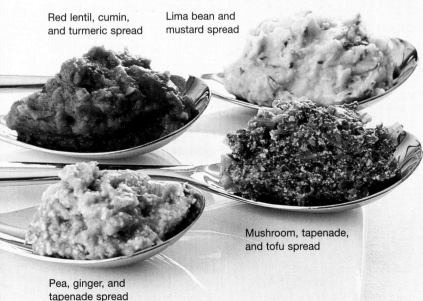

Mushroom, tapenade, and tofu spread

Pea, ginger, and tapenade spread

## Red lentil, cumin, and turmeric spread

ready in **25** minutes

1 tablespoon olive oil

1 onion (approx. 7oz/200g), finely chopped

1 garlic clove, chopped

1 bay leaf

2 teaspoons turmeric

2 teaspoons curry powder

½ teaspoon chili paste

2 teaspoons black mustard seeds

½ teaspoon cumin seeds

1 can red lentils (approx. 5oz/150g) drained and rinsed

10 fl oz (300ml) vegetable stock (*see p.149*)

1–2 tablespoons finely chopped fresh cilantro

Freshly ground black pepper, to taste

Heat the olive oil over medium-low heat in a heavy-bottomed saucepan and add the onion, garlic, and bay leaf. Cook gently until the onion is soft but not colored.

Stir in the turmeric, curry powder, chili paste, mustard seeds, and cumin and continue cooking gently for 3–4 minutes to allow the onion to absorb the flavors. Add the lentils and the stock. Stir, bring to a boil, reduce the heat, and simmer very gently for about 15 minutes, until the lentils are very tender and the stock is absorbed.

When cooking is complete, leave the lentils in the pan to cool a little, then mash them very coarsely. Stir in the cilantro and black pepper.

## Lima bean and mustard spread

ready in **20** minutes

1 bag (approx. 10oz/300g) frozen baby lima beans, thawed

Approx. 10fl oz (300ml) vegetable stock (*see p.149*)

2 tablespoons olive oil

1 heaped teaspoon Dijon mustard

2–3 tablespoons chopped parsley

Freshly ground black pepper, to taste

Put the beans in a heavy-bottomed saucepan and pour in enough vegetable stock to cover. Bring to a boil, cover the pan, reduce the heat, and simmer for about 15–20 minutes, until the beans have softened. Drain, setting aside the stock.

Put the hot beans in a bowl and add the olive oil and mustard. Mash the mixture with a fork or a potato masher until it is quite smooth. Stir in the chopped parsley, pepper, and more olive oil, if necessary, to loosen the mixture. If the spread still seems too stiff, stir in a little of the reserved stock.

## Mushroom, tapenade, and tofu spread

ready in **15** minutes

2 tablespoons olive oil

½ onion (approx. 2oz/60g), very finely chopped

2oz (50g) tofu, very finely chopped

5oz (150g) well-flavored mushrooms, such as brown mushrooms, field mushrooms, exotic mushrooms, or a mixture

2 rounded teaspoons black olive tapenade (*see p.148*)

Juice of ½ lemon

Freshly ground black pepper, to taste

1 tablespoon snipped chives

Heat the oil in a heavy-bottomed saucepan over medium heat, add the onion, and cook until the onion is softened but not colored. Add the tofu and cook, stirring, for 2–3 minutes. Add the mushrooms, stir well, and allow to cook gently for about 5 minutes, or until the mushrooms are soft. Stir in the tapenade, lemon juice, and some black pepper. Add the chives.

---

### SERVING IDEAS

**For a snack** Choose your favorite spread and top two rice cakes with it as a perfect snack.

**For lunch** Use your favorite spread as a filling for a small baked potato with a green salad on the side, or as an accompaniment to any protein.

**For dinner** Choose a spread, make it thinner with a little olive oil or yogurt and use it as a sauce to be eaten with grilled fish or chicken.

# Dips and sauces

A great way of using leftovers, these recipes can be served cold as a dip with crudités or as a topping for rice cakes or crackers, but can also be used to liven up a main meal. The red pesto is a fantastic pasta sauce and equally good on roasted vegetables. Each recipe serves two.

## SERVING IDEAS

**For a snack** Spread some of the lima beans with pepper and sun-dried tomato sauce on an oatcake.

**For lunch** Red pesto makes a great pasta sauce—eat with a side salad *(see pp.120–21)*.

**For dinner** Try the pepper and sun-dried tomato sauce hot with grilled fish or as a sauce with stir-fried tofu.

## Fish dip

| ready in | **5** | minutes |
|---|---|---|

2oz (60g) cold cooked fish

2 tablespoons low-fat cream cheese

2 tablespoons lemon juice

¼ teaspoon anchovy paste (optional)

1 tablespoon finely chopped fresh dill

Put all the ingredients in a bowl and mash them roughly together with a fork. Store in the fridge for up to three days.

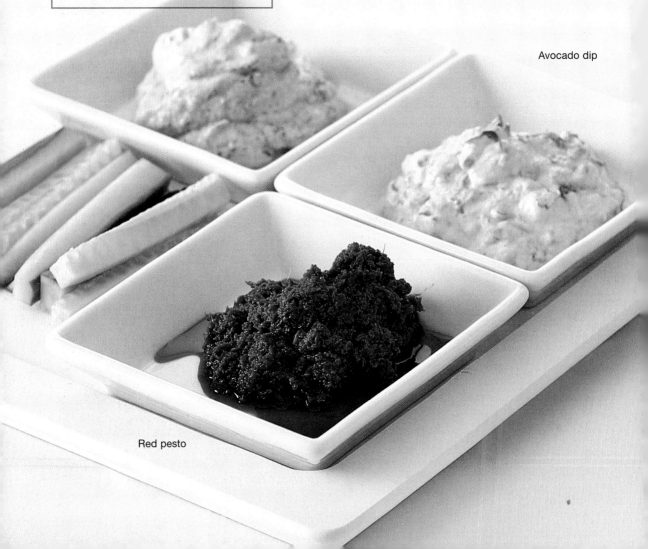

Fish dip

Avocado dip

Red pesto

## Avocado dip

ready in **5** minutes

½ avocado, pitted, peeled, and roughly chopped

2 tablespoons plain yogurt

1 tablespoon lime juice

1 tablespoon finely chopped cilantro

½ teaspoon grated fresh ginger

Put all the ingredients in a bowl and mash well with a fork. Top with some pine nuts for additional protein.

Cover the bowl with plastic wrap and put in the fridge until needed. It will keep, if refridgerated, for up to three days.

## Red pesto

ready in **10** minutes

1 jar (approx. 8oz/250g) sun-dried tomatoes in oil, drained

¼lb (125g) pine nuts

¼ pint (150ml) olive oil

Juice of ½ lemon

1 garlic clove

Freshly ground black pepper, to taste

Leaves from 1 small bunch parsley

Place all the ingredients in a blender or food processor and blend until fairly smooth. Pour into a container with a lid and store in the refrigerator. It will keep for up to four days.

## Pepper and sun-dried tomato sauce

ready in **10** minutes

1 jar (approx. 8oz/250g) mixed peppers in oil, drained

1 jar (approx. 8oz/250g) sun-dried tomatoes in oil, drained

5 tablespoons olive oil

Juice of ½ lemon

Freshly ground black pepper, to taste

Put the peppers and sun-dried tomatoes in a blender. Add the oil and lemon juice and blend until the mixture is thick but not too smooth. Add black pepper to taste. Store in the fridge for up to a week.

## Lima beans with pepper and sun-dried tomato sauce

ready in **15** minutes

1 tablespoon olive oil

1 garlic clove, crushed

¼ cup (60g) pepper and sun-dried tomato sauce (*see above*)

3½fl oz (100 ml) water

1 bag (approx. 10oz/300g) frozen baby lima beans, thawed

Heat the oil over medium-low heat in a small, heavy-bottomed saucepan. Add the garlic and cook for a minute or two to release its flavor. Add the pepper sauce and water, then the beans. Increase the temperature and simmer the ingredients for about 5 minutes, until the sauce is thick and the beans have heated through.

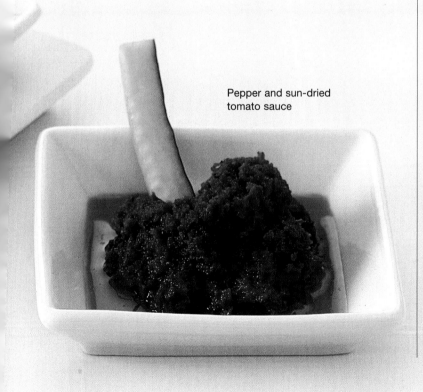

Pepper and sun-dried tomato sauce

# Lunch—the right proportions

Lunch can be a fresh cold salad prepared in minutes or a delicious cooked dish—as long as the food-group proportions fit the profile outlined below.

Cup both hands together with palms and fingers opened out showing 100% of their total surface area. This should give you an indication of how big your portion size should be. Your lunch should make up about 30% of your daily total food intake.

*100% of surface area of both hands*

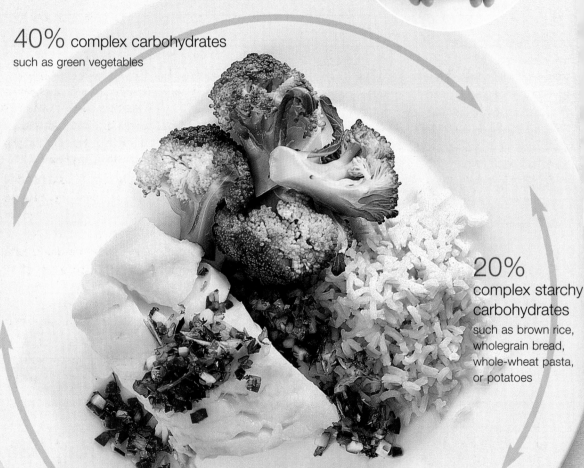

**40%** complex carbohydrates
such as green vegetables

**20%**
complex starchy
carbohydrates
such as brown rice,
wholegrain bread,
whole-wheat pasta,
or potatoes

**40%** protein
such as fish, chicken,
tofu, or beans

# Lunch and dinner

Serial dieters will know all too well that main meals can be an area fraught with difficulty. There is a general fear of overeating, but following The Food Doctor plan helps prepare you for main meals by ensuring that you are not overly hungry when you eat, and by giving you a clear idea of portion size too.

The ratios for protein and complex carbohydrates for lunch and dinner (see *opposite and p.72–73*) are both 40:60, although for lunch 20% of those complex carbohydrates are from starchy sources such as potatoes or brown rice. Using your hands as a simple guide to the size of the protein portion is easy: it is just under one "hand's-worth" (40% of the total surface area of both hands).

## A perfect lunch

Lunch is often eaten at work or at home between commitments or appointments. It doesn't have to be time-consuming, however (see *pp.36–37*). Making extra food the night before is my first choice for a convenient lunch. If you cook at home in the evening, simply make enough to take to work, or leave in the fridge for the next day's lunch. If you don't have any leftovers, then just make sure you have some basic ingredients to throw together—see my suggestions for recipes and menus (see *pp.76–77, 82–83*).

If you have a sandwich, choose one that has a complete protein filling, such as tuna, shrimp, chicken, or turkey. Sandwiches are by their nature higher in carbohydrates than I would ideally like you to have, but if you take a look at pages 82–83 you can see how easy it is to make them into more appropriate bases for an ideal Food Doctor meal. You aren't obliged to eat the sandwich alone, either: If you feel that it is lacking in protein, then you could add a handful of mixed nuts and seeds to redress the balance.

Many stores offer prepared salads, which are a great base for lunch. Often the protein is lacking, however, so if you get a pre-made tuna salad, then perhaps buy a small extra can of tuna as well and add it in.

If possible, don't buy lunch out every day since you won't have the same level of control that you have if you make something yourself. Once again, however, this doesn't mean complicated menus or hard work. You could do something as

## IDEAL PROTEIN CHOICES

These proteins are low in saturated fats and may contain beneficial essential fatty acids.

| | |
|---|---|
| Beans | Nuts (raw) |
| Chicken (skinless) | Seeds |
| Eggs | Tofu |
| Fish (especially oily fish) | Turkey (skinless) |
| Lentils | Veal |

## POOR PROTEIN CHOICES

Since these proteins are potential sources of trans or saturated fats, they are not ideal choices.

| | |
|---|---|
| Bacon | Lamb |
| Beef patties | Pheasant |
| Duck | Salami |
| Goose | Sausages |
| Ham | Soft cheese |

simple as open a can of tuna, mix in some chopped fresh dill or parsley, and eat the mixture with slices of sweet pepper, a few salad greens, and a slice of whole-wheat bread. Your meal doesn't have to be complicated or time-consuming to prepare—have whatever you feel like eating, as long as you keep the food group ratios in mind.

On the assumption that you ate breakfast at around 8am and a snack around 10:30am or so, lunch will probably be around 1pm. I suggest that you try and eat earlier rather than later. This will help you make better food decisions and not leave you in a position where your blood-glucose levels are very low, which will lead to hunger and cravings. Eating later makes you more likely to make poor food choices. The same applies in the evening: Aim to eat at about 7–7:30pm if possible, having had a midafternoon snack at approximately 4pm.

## Dinner-time

When it comes to preparing an evening meal, all too often clients tell me "I don't have time" or "I don't get in until late." I am not unsympathetic to the time issue—I work long hours too—but in order to achieve your goals you must look at the importance you have given to food in the past. If you usually rely on ready-made meals—the heat-and-eat sort of thing—then you must ask yourself how much this has played a part in your weight gain. Most ready-made meals have much higher fat and sugar levels than you might expect

and also, since protein usually costs more than carbohydrates, the meal costs are minimized if protein is limited.

When I discuss cooking with clients, I think there is a misconception that it requires a huge amount of time, and that's simply not the case. If you look at the recipes in this book you will see that many take just ten minutes to prepare, and others only a little longer. There is minimal effort in most of them, and I have tried to ensure that they are more like assembling or preparing food rather than "serious" cooking.

Occasionally I hear from clients that The Food Doctor plan for the evening meal doesn't quite satisfy them: If so, I suggest that, rather than eating more at dinner, or eating something sweet and sugary afterward, take a break for an hour or so, and then have a very small snack, once again with protein and vegetables. This could be some crudités and dip, or tuna with some lettuce leaves. It may not be traditional, but it works, and encourages sustainable and healthy weight loss.

## What to drink with your meal

I love wine. Drinking a glass or two at dinner is a real pleasure, and alcohol is not forbidden on The Food Doctor plan as long as you follow the rules (see p.145). If you choose not to drink alcohol, avoid juices and sodas, since they are sweetened and caffeinated. Water is best, whether sparkling or still, plain, or flavored with a slice of lemon, lime, or whatever you like, as long as it's sugar-free.

### IDEAL VEGETABLE CHOICES

There are so many good vegetable choices, but these ones have some of the lowest GI values.

| | | | |
|---|---|---|---|
| Eggplant | 10 | Onions | 10 |
| Cabbage | 10 | Red sweet peppers | 10 |
| Broccoli | 10 | Spinach | 10 |
| Lettuce | 10 | Tomatoes | 10 |
| Mushrooms | 10 | Carrots (raw) | 35 |

### POOR VEGETABLE CHOICES

Their high GI ratings make these vegetables relatively poor choices for your meal.

| | | | |
|---|---|---|---|
| Parsnips | 97 | Pumpkin | 75 |
| Potatoes (chips) | 95 | Turnips | 70 |
| Potatoes (mashed) | 90 | Potatoes (baked) | 65 |
| Carrots (cooked) | 85 | Beets | 64 |
| Fava beans | 80 | Potatoes (boiled) | 62 |

# Dinner—the right proportions

For your evening meal, 60% of your food should be based on vegetables but, unlike at lunch, you should avoid starchy complex carbohydrates, such as grains and potatoes.

Cup both hands together with your palms and fingers opened out showing 100% of their total surface area. This will give you an indication of how big your portion size should be. Your evening meal should make up about 30% of your daily total food intake.

100% of surface area of both hands

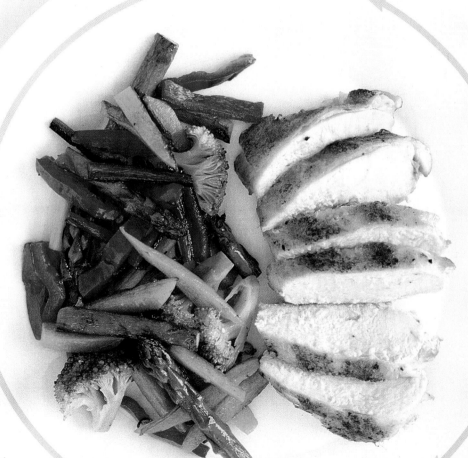

**40%**
protein
such as eggs, fish, tofu, beans, or lean meat

**60%** complex carbohydrates
such as a selection of vegetables

# Menu ideas

# Lunch or dinner

Although your lunch and dinner will be about the same size, the proportions of the food groups will differ slightly. These ideas show you how easy it is to make the ratios work.

## Chicken

- **chicken**  one portion of a simple chicken dish such as Cajun-spiced chicken or Indian spicy chicken (*see pp.130–31*), or chicken in summer herbs (*see p.123*) or coconut chicken (*see p.84*)

- **for lunch**  serve with a small baked potato or a few new potatoes, and a small portion of steamed green vegetables

  or

- **for dinner**  serve with a large portion of steamed green vegetables

## Eggs

- **eggs**  two eggs cooked as an omelet, or a frittata, for example—either simply seasoned or cooked with a delicious filling (*see pp.58, 86–87, 140*)

  and

- **for lunch**  serve with a chunk of wholegrain bread and a green salad, or a mixed side-salad (*see pp.112–13*)

  or

- **for dinner**  serve with a large portion of side-salad, or a large green salad and tomatoes

## Soup

- **soup**  one portion of (preferably home-made) soup, such as shrimp and watercress (*see p.101*) or vegetable and bean (*see p.103*)

  and

- **for lunch**  serve with wholegrain bread and perhaps a green salad

  or

- **for dinner**  add extra vegetables to the soup or serve with a side-salad

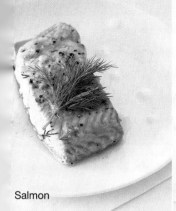

Salmon

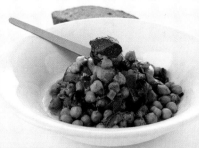

Chickpea and ratatouille stew

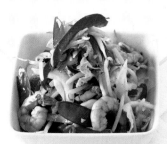

Shrimp and sweet chili stir-fry

## Fish

■ **fish**  one portion of grilled or poached fish, such as salmon or flounder, or a portion of a recipe such as seared cod (*see p.89*), shrimp and sweet chili stir-fry (*see p.108*), or swordfish with coriander and lime (*see p.98*)

and

■ **for lunch**  serve with a portion of brown rice or a few new potatoes, and a small portion of grilled vegetables

or

■ **for dinner**  serve with a large portion of grilled vegetables over a mixed leaf salad: drizzle over a tangy dressing (*see pp.128–29*)

## Beans

■ **beans**  one portion of a pulse-based dish, such as feta, tomato, and bean stir-fry (*see p.109*), chickpea and ratatouille stew (*see p.137*), or lima beans Italian-style (*see p.132*)

and

■ **for lunch**  serve with buckwheat noodles or brown rice

or

■ **for dinner**  increase the proportion of complex carbohydrates a little by adding a few extra vegetables to your dish

## Tofu

■ **tofu**  one portion of any tofu dish, such as leeks in red pesto and tofu sauce (*see p.106*), or green and white salad (*see p.113*)

and

■ **for lunch**  serve with brown rice and steamed green vegetables

or

■ **for dinner**  serve with a large portion of steamed green vegetables

# Menu ideas

# Packed lunch

Many of us do not have access to a kitchen during the day, so lunch needs to be either prepared in advance or very simple to put together. Here are some ideas.

## Cheese salad

- **cheese** a small handful of cheese, such as mozarella, cottage cheese, or goat cheese

  and

- **salad** a mixture of any fresh ingredients, such as half an avocado, a carrot, a large handful of salad greens, and a few olives

  and

- **bread** one large slice of wholegrain, rye, or gluten-free bread

## Healthy sandwich

- **protein filling** either one sliced egg flavored with herbs, a tablespoon of cottage cheese, or two slices of chicken, turkey, or smoked salmon

  and

- **bread** two slices of whole-wheat, rye, or gluten-free bread

  and

- **salad** a handful of salad greens and a few slices of tomato

## Rice salad with chicken

- **chicken** a small portion of grilled chicken (perhaps leftovers from the previous night's meal or a barbecue)

  and

- **rice salad** a few tablespoons of brown rice mixed with dressing (*see pp.114–15*) and two tablespoons of grilled vegetables, such as asparagus, broccoli, leeks, string beans, or an equivalent amount of raw chopped vegetables such as tomatoes, cucumbers, red sweet peppers, and scallions

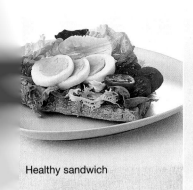

Healthy sandwich

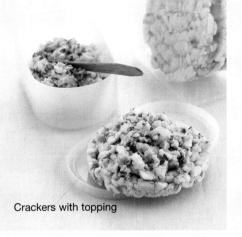

Crackers with topping

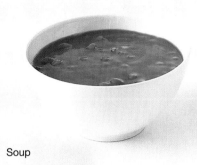

Soup

## Topped rice cakes

- **topping**  any protein-based topping, such as two boiled eggs chopped with mixed herbs, cottage cheese with chopped scallions and cucumber, or fish topping (*see pp.37, 68*)

  and

- **crackers**  two crackers, such as rice cakes, or crispbreads

  and

- **vegetables**  a few cherry tomatoes, for example, or some carrots, sweet peppers, or cucumber strips

## Pasta salad

- **fish**  a small portion of fish, such as smoked salmon, or canned tuna

  and

- **pasta**  a small portion of whole-wheat or buckwheat pasta or noodles

  and

- **salad vegetables**  a large handful of mixed vegetables, such as a scallions, a small sweet pepper, two tomatoes, two mushrooms, and a quarter of a zucchini

## Soup with fresh bread

- **soup**  one portion of (preferably home-made) soup, such as smoked fish chowder (*see p.85*), tomato and red pepper soup with cannellini beans (*see p.99*), or very quick gazpacho (*see p.101*)

  and

- **bread**  one thick slice of bread, such as wholegrain, rye, or gluten-free bread

# Menu ideas

# Quick meals

Possibly the most common excuse I hear is that eating healthy takes too much time. Here are six great ideas to dispel that myth. Vary the ingredients and start experimenting.

### Stir-fry

- **protein**   one portion of chicken, turkey, or fish, cut into strips, or shrimp, tofu cubes, or beans: If you wish, you could follow a stir-fry recipe such as chicken and cashew (*see p.102*), or feta, tomato, and bean (*see p.109*)

  and

- **vegetables**   if you're not following one of the recipes above, add a large handful of mixed chopped vegetables to your protein choice, such as bok choi, spinach, sweet peppers, snow peas, mushrooms, and beansprouts

  and (if lunch-time)

- **noodles**   a small portion of buckwheat noodles

### Frittata with salad greens

- **frittata**   choose from one of my frittata recipes, such as mushroom and tomato (*see p.58*), leek, Mediterranean, red pesto and sweet potato and dill (*see pp.86–87*)

  and

- **salad leaves**   a generous handful of mixed salad greens, such as watercress, arugula, red chard, and baby spinach

  and (if lunch-time)

- **baked potato**   one small baked potato

### Salmon with steamed vegetables

- **salmon**   one fillet simply poached or grilled, livened up with a marinade such as yogurt and ginger (*see p.127*), or cooked according to a recipe such as lime and dill salmon or coconut and coriander salmon (*see p.124–25*)

  and

- **vegetables**   a large portion of steamed vegetables, such as broccoli, cauliflower, snow peas, green beans, kale, spinach, asparagus, cabbage, carrots, and baby corn cobs

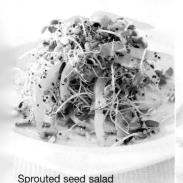

Sprouted seed salad

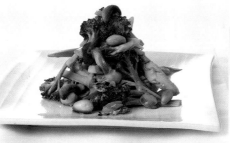

Chicken and cashew stir-fry

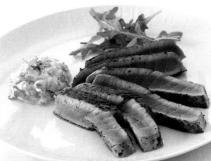

Cinnamon seared tuna

## Filled wrap

- **pancake wrap**  one buckwheat wrap (*see p.104*)

  and

- **protein filling**  make your own filling from food you have available, or try recipes such as avocado and scallop (*see p.105*), smoked salmon and poached egg (*see p.59*), or wild mushroom and prosciuitto (*see p.104*)

  and

- **salad**  if using a plain protein filling, such as cheese or grilled chicken, either add a side-salad such as avocado and watercress salad (*see p.120*), or put a handful of salad greens and tomato slices into the wrap

## Seared tuna with side dish

- **seared tuna**  a fresh tuna steak, seared in cinnamon or other spices (*see p.128*), or marinated in one of the marinade recipes, such as horseradish and lime or sesame oil and grainy mustard (*see p.126–27 for all recipes*)

  and

- **side-dish**  a portion of a vegetable-based side-dish such as ratatouille, onion and tomato niçoise, baby beets in horseradish, or stir-fried vegetables (*see p.96–97 for all recipes*)

  and (if lunch-time)

- **mashed potato**  a tablespoon of mashed potato

## Salad plate

- **salad**  choose from the recipes which contain a suitable protein serving, such as sprouted seed salad (*see p.119*), green and white salad (*see p.113*), avocado and quinoa salad (*see p.93*), or caesar salad (*see p.116*)

  and (if lunch-time)

- **potatoes or couscous**  a few new potatoes drizzled with walnut oil, or a small portion of couscous, brown rice, or bulgar wheat

# Delicious dinners...

Applying The Food Doctor principles to a main meal is simple: Just remember the ratios (*see pp.70–75*) and you can't go wrong.

## The usual choice

**Grilled lamb chop with roasted vegetables** This is a delicious way to eat vegetables, especially with herbs such as rosemary. The ratio of protein to carbohydrate is also fine, but the choice of meat could be better.

**Seared tuna with mashed potatoes and steamed asparagus** These foods are all healthy, nutritious, and good Food Doctor choices. Mashed potatoes are a traditional and comforting favorite and, if this meal were to be eaten at lunchtime, it would be fine. However there is a rule prohibiting eating starchy carbohydrates: Don't do it after 7pm.

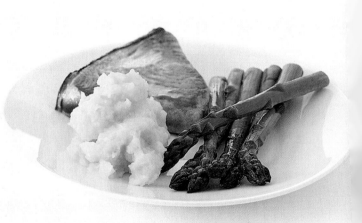

**Vegetable stir-fry with avocado and watercress salad** Stir-fries and salads are great ways of eating a wide variety of vegetables with all their nutrients still intact. They are also quick options. However, there is something missing this that stops this from being a whole and healthy meal.

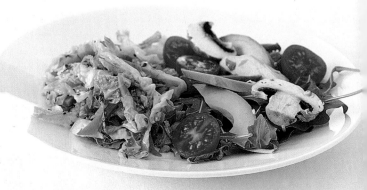

# can be diet friendly too

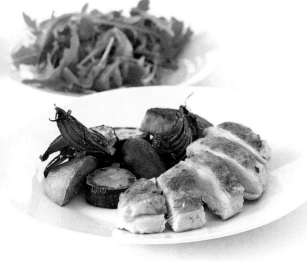

## The Food Doctor choice

Although grilling is a healthy option, a lamb chop is a relatively fatty choice. Red meat contains a higher amount of saturated fats than white meat.

- A grilled chicken breast has a much lower saturated fat content than lamb. Chicken is versatile and can easily be spiced up too (*see pp.130–131*).

- There is a wide range of fish available and many choices have the added bonus of being rich essential fats. Try red or gray mullet, sardines, or swordfish—either grilled or baked.

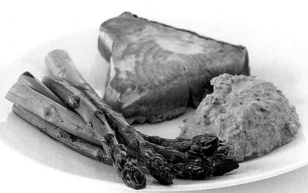

To make this the perfect evening meal, substitute Pea and ginger spread (*see p.66*) for the starchy mashed potatoes.

- Try some of the other delicious spreads (*see pp.66–67*). They all contain some protein too, so remember that when gauging portion sizes and ensure you have enough complex carbohydrate.

- Instead of the pea spread, you could try some steamed green vegetables a vegetable side dishes (*see pp.96–97 for examples*). As long as the protein:Complex carbohydrate ratio is right, feel free to experiment.

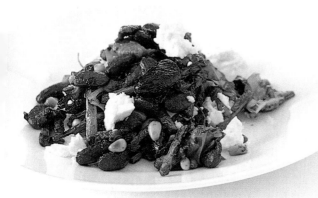

The missing element from the dinner on the left is protein. Without it, you won't be receiving the slow-release glucose it contains and you may find yourself hungry again before bedtime.

- The Feta, tomato, and bean stir-fry (*see p.109*) is a delicious alternative. The feta, pine nuts, and kidney beans together provide the needed protein.

- Another option might be to have a salad that has a protein element, such as the Avocado and quinoa (*see p.93*) or Root vegetable and goat cheese (*see p.112*).

# Lunch on the run ...

Good intentions are all very well, but what happens when you're buying lunch to go? Remember the ratios and you can easily create a healthy option.

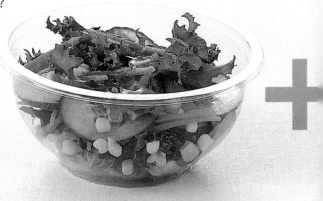

## The usual choice

**Salad** How can you go wrong with a salad? Well, if you just eat a plain green salad, you're missing out on essential food groups and not fueling your body properly. Add some protein to complete the ratio of foods.

**Sandwich** Surely a sandwich packed with salad greens is a healthy option? No, since it lacks a good balance of protein and complex carbohydrates. By adding extra filling or removing one layer of bread from your sandwich, you can redress the ratio of food groups and turn your sandwich into a healthy choice.

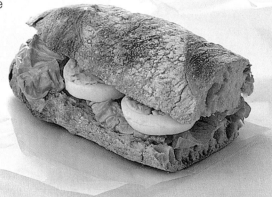

**Vegetable soup and a roll**
This is an excellent choice for a perfect lunch on the run—if you choose the right foods in the right proportions. This choice needs additional protein and fiber to turn it into the perfect meal.

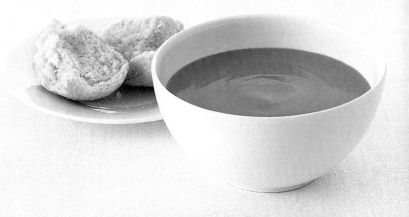

# making it healthier

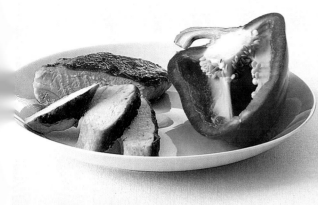

## The Food Doctor choice

A salad can be a very smart choice if you know your vegetables. Eat those that are rich in vitamin C and other antioxidants, such as red sweet peppers, raw carrots, watercress, tomatoes, and try to vary your choices to make sure you get a range of nutrients.

- Add a brown rice salad: It is high in B vitamins, so it's a good choice for a lunchtime starchy complex carbohydrate.

- Protein such as chicken or tuna boosts the mineral content of your meal and makes it convert more slowly into glucose.

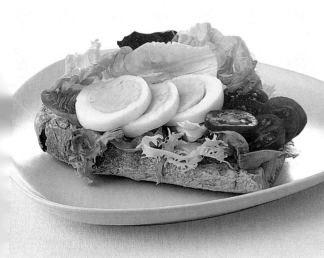

White bread is a poor choice because it is low in fiber, and thus has a high GI value (see p.21). Instead, try rye bread, since it is dense and allows you to vary your grain intake, or sourdough (in general, I believe we eat more yeast products than we should).

- Add tomato for extra fiber and antioxidants.

- Chicken, tuna, egg, or smoked salmon are all good sources of protein for sandwich fillings.

- Remember to minimize mayonnaise and butter. Use seasonings instead: A layer of mustard on the bread adds flavor and a moist texture.

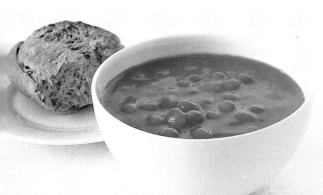

Opt for vegetable-based soups over those based on cream or potatoes, and just add fiber and protein to make soup a smart option.

- Add some chickpeas or other beans to boost the protein ratio of your soup, or add some tofu, shredded ham, or sliced chicken breast.

- Stir in a small can of corn or some baby spinach leaves to give your soup extra fiber.

- Swap the white roll for whole-wheat or rye to avoid high-GI refined flour products.

# Coconut chicken

The spices and coconut give flavor to the chicken, which can be prepared without the rice for an even quicker meal with vegetables or salad. Serves two.

**ready in 30 minutes**

1 boneless, skinless chicken breast (approx. ¼lb/150g)

1 cup (250ml) coconut milk

½ teaspoon chili paste

1–2 tablespoons chopped fresh cilantro

1 garlic clove, crushed

Freshly ground black pepper, to taste

1½ cups (350ml) vegetable stock (*see p.149*)

½ cup (150g) brown rice

1 teaspoon olive oil

1 small red pepper, cored, seeded, and cut into strips

Cut the chicken breast into strips. Place the coconut milk, chili paste, cilantro, garlic, and black pepper in a bowl and mix well. Add the chicken strips and stir them into the mixture. Set aside to marinate while cooking the rice.

Bring the stock to the boil in a heavy-bottomed saucepan, add the rice, and cover. Return to a boil, then reduce the heat and simmer for 25–30 minutes, or until the rice is cooked. Drain, stir in just a little olive oil and perhaps some chopped herbs, cover, and keep warm.

Heat a wok or frying pan over medium heat and pour in the chicken and the marinade. Cook gently for about 5 minutes, until the chicken is almost cooked. Add the red pepper strips and cook for a further 5 minutes, until the chicken is fully cooked but the pepper is still firm. Serve immediately.

## SERVING IDEAS

**For lunch** Serve exactly as the recipe suggests for a delicious lunch.

**For dinner** Omit the rice from the dish and in its place add a mixture of lightly steamed green vegetables. Or add finely chopped vegetables such as broccoli and zuchinni to the stir-fry.

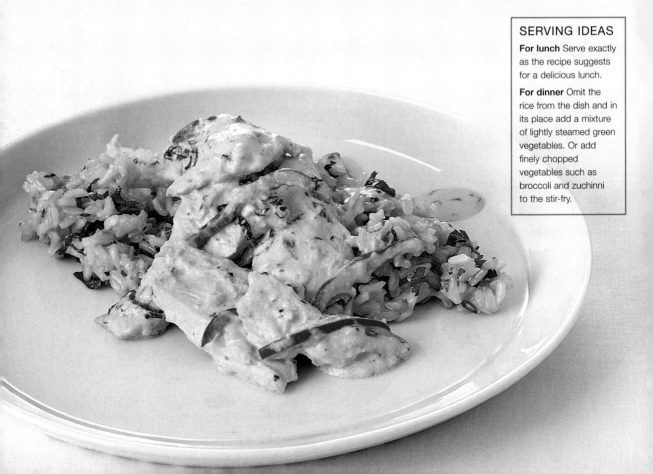

# Smoked fish chowder

LUNCH OR **DINNER**

Provided you use fresh (not frozen) fish, stock, and shrimp, you could make double the quantity of this recipe and freeze what you do not use. Serves two.

ready in 30 minutes

SERVING IDEAS

**For lunch** Serve with a slice of rye bread.

**For dinner** Try one of the side salads on pp.120–21 with this hearty soup, or stir in some steamed green vegetables.

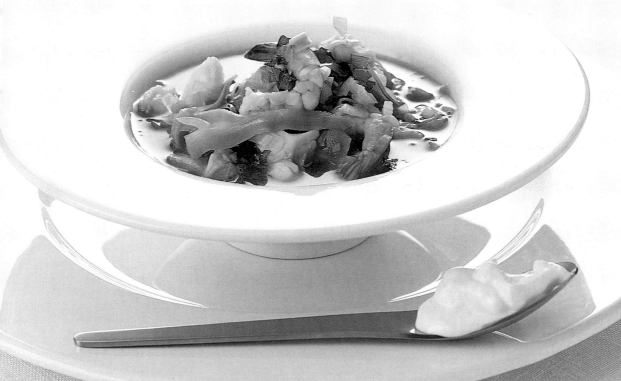

1 tablespoon olive oil

1 small leek, finely sliced

2 shallots, finely sliced

1 medium carrot, grated

1 pint (500ml) fish stock (*see p.149*)

2 tablespoons Thai fish sauce (optional)

1 tablespoon lemon juice

½lb (200g) smoked haddock, cod, or trout, skin removed and cut into chunks

2½oz (75g) cooked shrimp

Freshly ground black pepper, to taste

2–3 tablespoons plain yogurt

1 tablespoon chopped parsley

Heat the oil in a heavy-bottomed saucepan over medium heat, add the leek, shallots, and carrot and cook gently until softened. Pour in the fish stock, fish sauce, if using, and lemon juice. Bring to a boil, reduce the heat, and simmer for about 5 minutes.

Add the smoked fish and simmer for about 8 minutes until the fish is heated through. Add the shrimp and black pepper and simmer further until they are hot.

Put a generous tablespoon of plain yogurt in each of two soup bowls, divide the hot chowder between the two, then stir and top with the parsley.

# Frittatas

These frittatas are filling and a good vegetarian option. Each frittata can be eaten either still warm from cooking or cold with some salad. If you aren't sharing your frittata, save the other half for snacks throughout the day. Each recipe serves two.

Mediterranean frittata

## Mediterranean frittata

ready in **15** minutes

1 tablespoon olive oil

1 onion (approx. 3½oz/100g) sliced

½ red pepper, cored, seeded, and diced

½ green pepper, cored, seeded, and diced

2 medium tomatoes, sliced

4 eggs

2 tablespoons plain yogurt

2 tablespoons water

1 teaspoon dried mixed herbs

Freshly ground black pepper, to taste

8 black olives, pitted

Heat the oil in a skillet over medium heat and add the onion and diced peppers. Cook gently until softened. Add the tomatoes and cook for another 2–3 minutes.

Break the eggs into a bowl and add the yogurt, water, herbs, and black pepper to taste. Mix the ingredients together well. Pour the mixture over the vegetables in the pan, stirring gently to help the egg mixture get under the vegetables. Scatter the olives evenly over the top. Cook the frittata very gently until the bottom is firm and lightly brown. Be careful not to let it burn.

To cook the top, put the pan under a medium broiler for 4–5 minutes, until lightly browned.

## Leek frittata

ready in **20** minutes

1 tablespoon olive oil

Juice of 1 lemon

4 medium leeks, finely sliced

1 tablespoon cumin seeds

4 eggs

Freshly ground black pepper, to taste

2 tablespoons plain yogurt

Hard goat cheese or Manchego, finely grated

Heat the olive oil and lemon juice in a skillet, add the leeks and cook over moderate heat for 5–10 minutes or until soft.

While the leeks are cooking put the cumin seeds in a small pan and toss over high heat for a few seconds until they are just toasted.

Beat the eggs, black pepper, yogurt, and cumin seeds together, pour over the cooked leeks, and cook until the underside is set and golden (about 5 minutes).

Scatter the top with grated cheese. To cook the top, put the pan under a medium broiler for 4–5 minutes until it is golden.

## Sweet potato and dill frittata

ready in **25** minutes

1 small sweet potato (approx. ½lb/175g)

1 tablespoon olive oil

1 small onion sliced

4 eggs

2 tablespoons plain yogurt

2 tablespoons water

½ teaspoon turmeric

1 teaspoon dried dill or 1 tablespoon chopped fresh dill

Freshly ground black pepper, to taste

Simmer the sweet potato in its skin in gently boiling water for about 15 minutes or until just soft. When cooked, peel and slice it.

Heat the oil in a small skillet over medium-low heat. Add the onion and cook until softened. Break the eggs into a bowl and add the yogurt, water, turmeric, dill, and black pepper to taste. Whisk the egg mixture together well and pour over the onions in the pan. Add the sweet potato slices and spread evenly over the contents of the pan. Cook very gently until the underside of the frittata is firm and lightly browned.

To cook the top, put the pan under a medium broiler for about 5 minutes, watching carefully, until the frittata top is lightly browned.

## Red pesto frittata

ready in **20** minutes

4 eggs

¼ cup (60g) red pesto (*see p.69*)

2 tablespoons chopped fresh mint

3 tablespoons plain yogurt

Freshly ground black pepper, to taste

1 tablespoon olive oil

1 small onion, chopped

Break the eggs into a bowl and add the red pesto, mint, yogurt, and black pepper. Whisk everything together well.

Heat the oil in a skillet over medium heat, add the onion and cook until softened. Pour in the egg mixture and cook until the frittata is firm and the base is golden. Slide the pan under a medium broiler until the top of the frittata is cooked and golden.

### SERVING IDEAS

**For lunch** Serve with a few new potatoes and some chopped tomatoes and green leaves.

**For dinner** Serve with onion and tomato nicoise or one of the other side dishes on pp.96–97.

# Lemon spinach soup

The small dark French lentils give great flavor and texture to this soup. If they are not available canned, you could cook up some dried French lentils, or use ordinary green lentils instead. Serves two.

**ready in 20 minutes**

1 tablespoon olive oil

1 small onion, finely chopped

1 garlic clove, chopped

1 can (approx. 13oz/400g) French lentils, drained and rinsed

3 teaspoons bouillon powder

1 star anise

4 cups (1 liter) water

½ lb (8oz/250g) spinach, finely shredded

3 tablespoons lemon juice

Freshly ground black pepper

2 tablespoons plain yogurt

Heat the olive oil over medium-low heat in a small saucepan, add the onion and garlic, and cook until softened. Set aside.

Put the lentils in a heavy-bottomed saucepan, stir in the bouillon powder, then add the star anise and water. Bring to a boil, reduce the heat, and simmer for 5–10 minutes. Add the shredded spinach and, when it is well wilted, stir in the onion and garlic mixture, lemon juice, and black pepper to taste.

Top with a good tablespoonful of yogurt in each bowl, and serve hot.

## SERVING IDEAS

**For lunch** Serve with a fresh whole-grain roll.

**For dinner** Everything you need is in this tasty soup, but if you would like something extra, stir in some steamed broccoli.

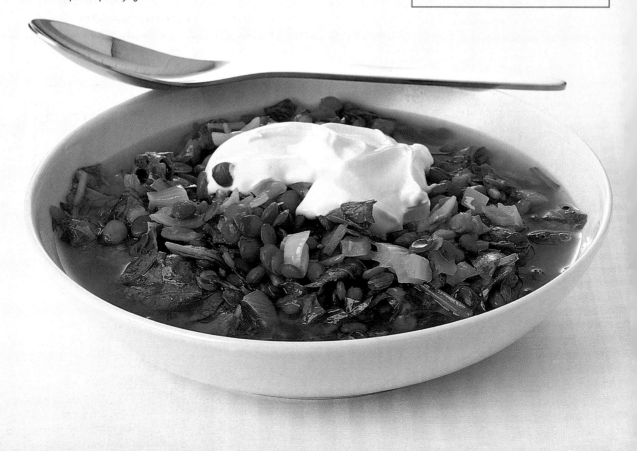

# Seared cod on spinach

The sweet-and-sour onion sauce turns simple cod into a superbly satisfying meal. You can substitute any other white fish if you prefer. Serves two.

**ready in 30 minutes**

2½ tablespoons olive oil, plus extra for brushing

1 small onion, finely sliced

1 teaspoon honey

½ cup (125ml) fish stock (*see p.149*)

1 tablespoon white wine vinegar

1 teaspoon soy sauce

1 teaspoon mustard

Few drops Thai fish sauce (optional)

2 thick cod fillets (approx. 7oz/150g each), skin on

½lb (8oz/250g) spinach

Freshly grated nutmeg, to taste

Put an oven-proof dish into a preheated oven at 400°F/200°C/gas mark 6.

To make the sauce, heat 2 tablespoons of oil in a heavy-bottomed pan over medium heat, add the onion, and cook until it has softened and is turning golden. Add the honey and cook for a further 10 minutes, or until the onion caramelizes. Add the fish stock and vinegar and simmer hard for 8–10 minutes to reduce the liquid by half. Stir in the soy sauce and mustard. Add a few drops of Thai fish sauce, if you wish.

While the sauce is reducing, cook the fish. Heat the remaining olive oil in a frying pan over a medium-high heat and cook the fillets skin side down for 3–4 minutes until the skin is crisp. Brush the top of the fish with a little oil.

Take the hot dish out of the oven and put in the fish, skin side up. Return the dish to the oven for about 5 minutes.

Steam the spinach in a steamer insert over a pan of simmering water until the leaves are just wilted. Sprinkle a little nutmeg over it and keep warm until the fish is ready. Serve with the onion sauce.

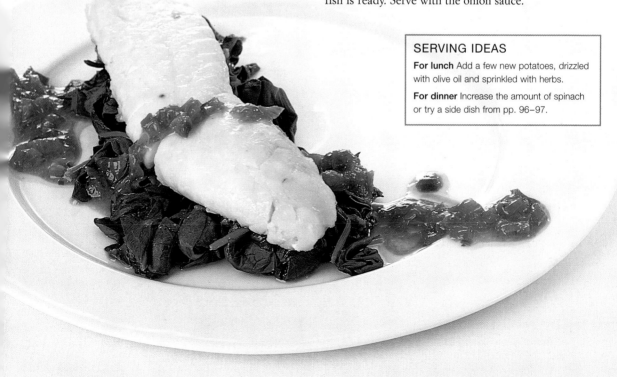

> ### SERVING IDEAS
>
> **For lunch** Add a few new potatoes, drizzled with olive oil and sprinkled with herbs.
>
> **For dinner** Increase the amount of spinach or try a side dish from pp. 96–97.

# Tomatoes stuffed with quinoa

**LUNCH OR DINNER**

The colorfully named beefsteak tomato is ideal for stuffing because it is large and has firm, thick flesh that will not collapse during cooking. Here, it is stuffed with well-flavored quinoa, and given crunch with the addition of pine nuts. Serves two.

**ready in 30 minutes**

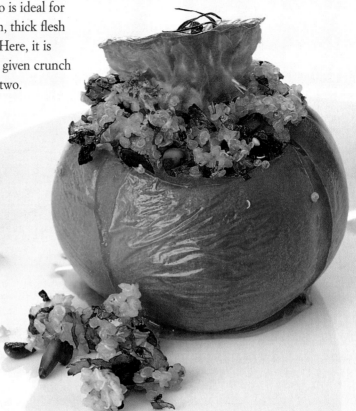

## SERVING IDEAS

**For lunch** Serve with a small baked potato and a green salad.

**For dinner** Cook up a little extra quinoa to serve on the side and eat with a side salad or some chopped, crunchy sweet peppers.

Approx. 1½ cups (250ml) vegetable stock (*see p.149*)

½ cup (100g) quinoa

2 beefsteak or other large tomatoes

Freshly ground black pepper

2 tablespoons olive oil

1 small onion (approx. ½ cup/100g), chopped

1 garlic clove, chopped

1 tablespoon lemon juice

Grated zest of ½ lemon

2 tablespoons pine nuts

1 tablespoon chopped fresh cilantro

2 tablespoons chopped fresh parsley

Heat the stock in a heavy-bottomed saucepan, add the quinoa, stir and simmer for 15 minutes, or until the quinoa is tender. If the stock has not been absorbed, drain the quinoa into a sieve.

While the quinoa is cooking, slice the tops off the tomatoes and scoop out and discard the seeds, taking care not to break through the pith and skin. Grind some pepper into the tomatoes. Preheat the oven to 180°C/350°F/gas mark 4.

Heat the oil in a heavy-bottomed saucepan, add the onion and garlic, and cook until golden. Add the drained quinoa, lemon juice and zest, pine nuts, and chopped herbs to the pan and mix well. Spoon the ingredients into the tomatoes and top with the "lids." Put the tomatoes in an oven-proof dish, cover, and cook in the oven for 15 minutes, or until the tomatoes are soft.

# Thai-style chicken

This dish is very simple to make, yet has a fresh exotic taste. Experiment with the herbs and spices to create different flavors. Serves two.

ready in **30** minutes

### SERVING IDEAS

**For lunch** Serve with brown rice. Add some chopped herbs for interest.

**For dinner** Try using extra carrots and celery to increase the meal size slightly, or add some fresh greens as an accompaniment.

1 boneless, skinless chicken breast (approx. 4oz/125g), sliced with the grain of the meat to make four equal-sized pieces

¼ cup (60ml) lemon juice, divided

Freshly ground black pepper, to taste

2 small leeks (approx. 5oz/150g when cleaned), finely sliced

½ cup (125g) grated carrots

2 sticks celery, halved and finely sliced lengthways

3 scallions, finely sliced lengthways

1 plump lemon grass stem, finely sliced

4 sprigs fresh thyme

1 cup (250ml) vegetable stock (*see p.149*)

2 tablespoons dry white wine (optional)

Put the chicken pieces in a bowl with half of the lemon juice and black pepper, mix well, and set aside to marinate while you prepare the vegetables.

Put the vegetables, herbs, and chicken in a shallow frying pan with a lid. Add the stock, white wine, if using, and the remaining lemon juice. Bring to a boil, cover the pan, reduce the heat, and simmer very gently for about 20–25 minutes, until the chicken is cooked and the vegetables are tender. Serve immediately.

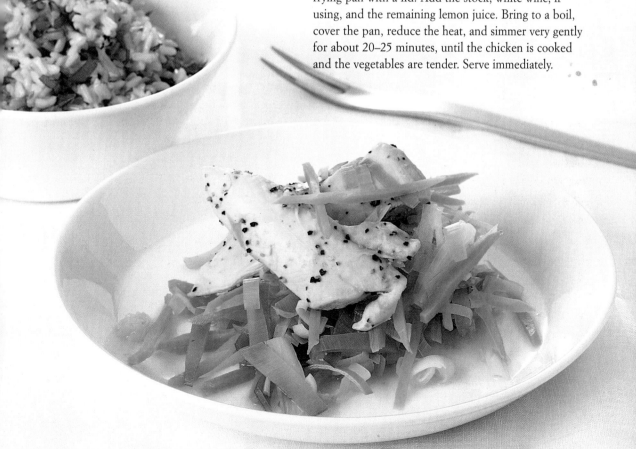

# Fish plaki

**LUNCH OR DINNER**

The tangy tomato sauce is tasty and thick, and thus very filling. This dish can also be made with chicken if that is what you have available. Serves two.

**ready in 30 minutes**

1 tablespoon olive oil, plus extra for greasing

1 slice whole-grain or rye bread, crumbed

1 can (approx. 7½oz/225g) chopped tomatoes

2 tablespoons chopped fresh parsley

1 garlic clove, crushed

1 pinch cayenne or chili pepper

Freshly ground black pepper, to taste

1 tablespoon lemon juice

¾ lb (350–400g) firm white fish fillets, such as cod, haddock, or orange roughy

Preheat the oven to 180°C/350°F/gas mark 4. Lightly oil an oven-proof dish.

Put the breadcrumbs, tomatoes, parsley, garlic, cayenne, black pepper, and lemon juice in a saucepan, bring to a boil, and simmer for a couple of minutes, stirring well.

Put the fish in the prepared dish, brush with the oil, and top with the sauce. Cover the dish with foil and bake in the preheated oven for about 20 minutes, depending on the thickness of the fillets, until the fish is cooked through but still moist. Serve at once.

## SERVING IDEAS

**For lunch** Serve with some brown rice and ratatouille (see p.96).

**For dinner** Try pairing this with a side dish on pp.96–97 or one of the spreads on pp.66–67.

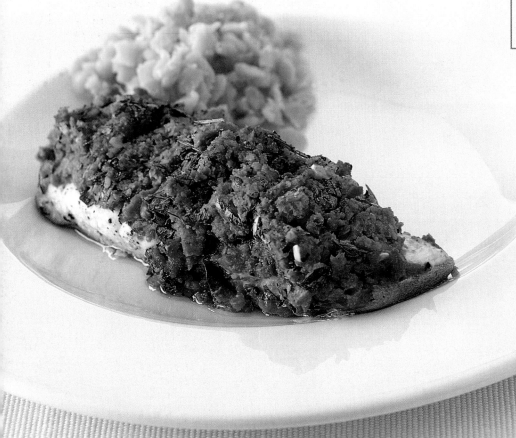

# Avocado and quinoa salad

This dish uses quinoa because it is a gluten-free grain that has a good protein content. Bulgar wheat or couscous are good substitutes. Serves two.

**ready in 30 minutes**

1 cup (250ml) vegetable stock (*see p.149*)

½ cup (125g) quinoa

2 eggs, hard-boiled

1 avocado

2 tablespoons lemon juice

2 scallions, trimmed and finely sliced

½ cup (100g) small, firm mushrooms (white, brown, or wild), cleaned and sliced

1 medium yellow pepper, cored, seeded, and cut into strips

6 black olives, pitted

Freshly ground black pepper

1 tablespoon chopped fresh cilantro

Olive oil, to drizzle

Heat the stock in a heavy-bottomed saucepan, pour in the quinoa, and simmer for about 20 minutes, until all the stock is absorbed.

While the quinoa is cooking, shell the eggs and slice them. Peel, halve, and slice the avocado (at the last minute, if possible) and sprinkle it with a little of the lemon juice so that it does not turn brown.

When the quinoa is cooked, stir in the remaining lemon juice and allow the quinoa to cool a little. Then gently fold in the remaining ingredients, drizzle with olive oil, and serve.

## SERVING IDEAS

**For lunch** This is already a very filling salad that can be served alone, but you could add a small baked potato.

**For dinner** This is a substantial dish, but you can add some extra chopped salad vegetables if you wish.

# Sauces, salsas, and compotes

These accompaniments are packed full of various tasty spices and herbs, making them ideal for brightening up any meal. They all serve two and, with the exception of the yogurt sauce with green herbs, can be stored in the refrigerator for a few days at a time.

## Green salsa

**ready in 15 minutes**

½ cucumber (about ¼ lb/100g)

1 kiwi, peeled, halved lengthways, and sliced

4 scallions, finely sliced

1 tablespoon olive oil

Juice of ½ lime

1 teaspoon crushed coriander seeds (or ground cilantro)

1 tablespoon chopped fresh cilantro

Freshly ground black pepper

½ teaspoon Thai green curry paste (optional)

Cut the cucumber, which should not be peeled, in quarters lengthways and slice off the angle to remove most of the seeds. Roughly chop the remaining cucumber pieces.

Place all the ingredients in a bowl, stir to mix them well, and leave to stand for 10 minutes before using.

## Orange and five-spice stir-fry sauce

**ready in 5 minutes**

1 tablespoon five-spice powder (*see p.148*)

Zest of 1 orange

½ cup (125ml) orange juice

Juice of 1 lemon

Freshly ground black pepper

Put all the ingredients in a bowl and mix together well. Use as a stir-fry sauce for portions of chicken, tofu cubes, fish, and mixed vegetables.

Red salsa

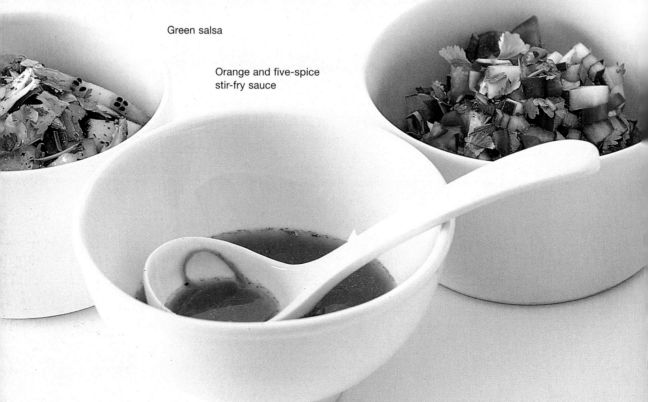

Green salsa

Orange and five-spice stir-fry sauce

# Red salsa

ready in **5** minutes

½ cucumber (about ¼lb/100g)

1 small red onion, finely chopped

2 medium tomatoes, chopped

1 red pepper, cored, seeded, and chopped

1 fresh red chili (optional), finely chopped

1 small cucumber, finely diced

2 tablespoons chopped fresh cilantro

1 tablespoon snipped chives

1 tablespoon lime juice

1 tablespoon olive oil

Freshly ground black pepper

Cut the cucumber, which should not be peeled, in quarters lengthways and cut the seeds away from the flesh. Roughly chop the remaining cucumber pieces.

Place all the ingredients in a bowl and mix well together. Add black pepper to taste. Sprinkle some sea salt over the salsa, if necessary. Serve immediately.

# Leek compote

ready in **20** minutes

2 small leeks, outer leaves removed, finely sliced

2 tablespoons olive oil

Grated zest of ½ lemon

Grated zest of ½ orange

1 teaspoon lemon juice

½ teaspoon soy sauce

Freshly ground black pepper

Freshly grated nutmeg, to taste

1 tablespoon plain yogurt

1 scallion, trimmed and finely sliced

Put the leeks in a wide heavy-bottomed saucepan with the olive oil and the grated zests. Heat gently, stirring occasionally, for about 15 minutes, or until the leeks are very soft and almost melted together. Stir in the lemon juice, soy sauce, nutmeg, and black pepper to taste. Add the yogurt and stir gently until the sauce is smooth. Stir in the sliced scallion. Serve warm, or leave to cool before serving.

# Yogurt sauce with green herbs

ready in **20** minutes

1 cup (250ml) plain yogurt

¼ lb (150g) mixed fresh arugula, watercress, spinach, and basil

2 tablespoons lemon juice

Grated zest of ½ lemon

½ cup olive oil

1 garlic clove

½ cup (100g) pine nuts

Put all the ingredients in a blender and mix together. To make things a little easier, the green leaves can be added to the blender in two or three batches, if preferred.

## SERVING IDEAS

**For lunch** The yogurt sauce with green herbs can be used over hot pasta with a good portion of grated goat cheese.

**For dinner** All the sauces work with chicken breasts or fish fillets, especially if they've been cooked on the grill.

Leek compote

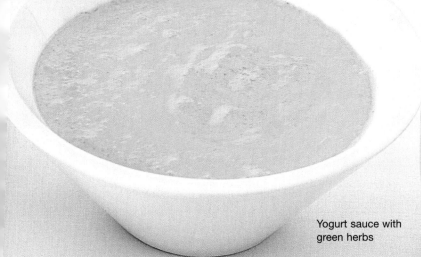

Yogurt sauce with green herbs

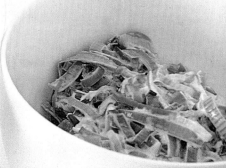

# Side dishes

These vegetable side dishes are perfect additions to any lunch or evening meal. Each tastes just as great hot or cold, so try one as a side dish with your dinner and save some to accompany your lunch or snack for the next day. Each recipe serves two.

## Ratatouille

ready in **30** minutes

Eggplant can be bitter, unless it has been salted. If you have time, slice it (reasonably thinly) and layer in a colander with a sprinkling of salt between layers. Leave for at least half an hour to remove the bitter juices. Rinse, drain, and pat dry.

¼ cup (60ml) olive oil

1 eggplant (approx. ½lb/250g), trimmed and sliced moderately thinly

2 zucchini (approx. ½lb/250g total weight), trimmed and sliced moderately finely

1 garlic clove, chopped

4 small tomatoes (approx. 10oz/300g total weight), roughly chopped

2 tablespoons chopped fresh parsley

Freshly ground black pepper, to taste

Heat the oil in a wide-bottomed saucepan over medium-low heat, add the sliced vegetables and the garlic, and cook gently for about 10 minutes, or until they are all soft and turning golden. Add the tomatoes and stir them down into the other ingredients. Stir in the parsley and black pepper to taste. Cover the pan and cook for an additional 15 minutes or so over medium heat, until all the vegetables are really soft and blended together. Stir occasionally to prevent sticking.

Note: This recipe also freezes well, so it is a good idea to make it in quantity. You can use this ratatouille in the chickpea and ratatouille stew (*see p.137*).

---

## SERVING IDEAS

**For lunch** Try the onion and tomato niçoise stirred into pasta with some chicken or fish and save a little to eat with cubed feta as a snack.

**For dinner** Any of these vegetable side dishes taste great with the various salmon fillet recipes on pp.124–25.

---

## Onion and tomato niçoise

ready in **30** minutes

2 tablespoons olive oil

2 onions (approx. ½lb/250g), halved lengthways and finely sliced

1 garlic clove, crushed

1 sprig fresh rosemary (or ½ teaspoon dried rosemary)

2 sprigs thyme (or 1 teaspoon dried thyme)

1 bay leaf

2 tomatoes (approx. ½lb/250g), sliced

12 black olives, pitted

6 anchovy fillets (washed if salted, drained if in oil), chopped

Freshly ground black pepper, to taste

Heat the oil in a large, heavy-bottomed saucepan over medium-low heat, add the onions, garlic, and herbs and cook gently for 20 minutes until soft and creamy. Add the tomatoes and cook for a couple of minutes until they soften, then stir in the olives and anchovy fillets. Add black pepper to taste and serve immediately.

Note: If you leave the saucepan on medium-low heat for an extra hour, the dish will be so mellowed that you will not be able tell the onions from the black olives.

# Baby beets in a horseradish sauce

ready in **15** minutes

4–6 baby beets (approx. ¾ lb/350g)

2oz (60g) soft silken tofu (or plain tofu)

2 tablespoons horseradish sauce (*see p.148*)

2 tablespoons lemon juice

Freshly ground black pepper, to taste

Leave the tops and tails on the beets and make sure the skin is intact. This will keep the color from leaching out of the beets as they cook. Boil them in very lightly salted water for about 25 minutes, or drizzle them with a tablespoon of olive oil and roast in an oven set to 350°F/180°C/gas mark 4 for about 25 minutes.

When the beets are cooked, slide off the skins, trim off the tops and tails, and cut into chunks.

To make the sauce, put the tofu, horseradish sauce, lemon juice, and black pepper into a blender and blend to make a smooth sauce with a creamy consistency, adding a little water if necessary. Heat the sauce in a pan and pour over the beets. Serve warm as a vegetable accompaniment or cold as a salad.

# Stir-fried vegetables

ready in **10** minutes

1 tablespoon caraway seeds

1 tablespoon olive oil

5oz (150g) green cabbage (coarse center stem removed), shredded

½ cup (100g) coarsely grated carrots

1 tablespoon lemon juice

Heat a wok or frying pan over medium-high heat. Put in the caraway seeds and dry-roast them for 2–3 minutes. Add the olive oil and vegetables to the pan, and stir to cover the vegetables with the oil. Add the lemon juice and stir-fry for about 5 minutes, until the vegetables are heated through.

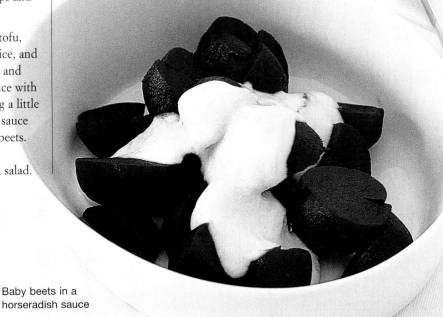

Baby beets in a horseradish sauce

# Swordfish with coriander and lime

Try this recipe with tuna in place of swordfish; both provide dense, meaty steaks. Try grilling these in the summer instead of frying. Serves two.

ready in **20** minutes

2 teaspoons coriander seeds

2 teaspoons fennel seeds

1 lime, halved

2 swordfish steaks (approx. 5oz/150g each)

Freshly ground black pepper, to taste

1 tablespoon olive oil

Put the coriander and fennel seeds on a cutting board and crush with the bottom of a heavy pan until fine, or use a spice grinder. Squeeze the lime halves over the steaks and season with black pepper. Sprinkle the ground seeds over the steaks and press them in well. Put the steaks aside for about 5 minutes for the flavors to be absorbed by the fish.

Heat the oil in a frying pan over medium heat. Put in the fish steaks and cook each side for about 4 minutes. The steaks should be just cooked through and golden on the outside. Serve immediately.

## SERVING IDEAS

**For lunch** Red salsa (*see p.94*) with a few spoonfuls of brown rice or couscous makes a tasty lunchtime accompaniment.

**For dinner** Serve with vegetable stir-fry or another side dish from pp.96–97.

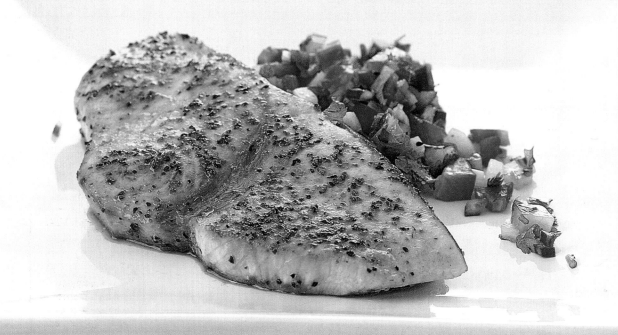

# Tomato and red pepper soup with cannellini beans

**LUNCH** OR **DINNER**

The beans can be swapped for most other pulses, depending on what you have available. The soup freezes well so try making it in bulk. Serves two.

ready in **20** minutes

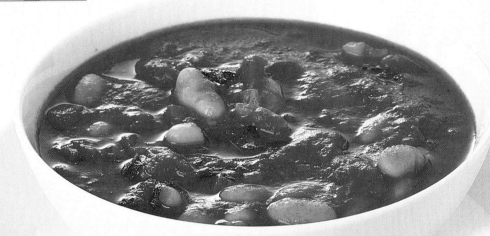

1 tablespoon olive oil

1 small onion, finely chopped

1 garlic clove, finely chopped

1 large red pepper, cored, seeded and chopped

1 can (13oz/400g) chopped tomatoes

1 tablespoon tomato purée

½ teaspoon paprika

1 large sprig fresh thyme (or ½ teaspoon dried thyme)

1 can (13oz/400g) cannellini beans

2 cups (17fl oz/500ml) vegetable stock (*see p.149*)

Handful fresh basil leaves, shredded, to garnish

Heat the olive oil in a heavy-bottomed saucepan over medium heat, add the onion, garlic, and red pepper, and cook until softened but not colored.

Add the remaining ingredients. Bring the mixture to a boil, reduce the heat, and simmer gently for 15 minutes. Garnish with the basil leaves before serving.

## SERVING IDEAS

**For lunch** Serve with a slice of whole-wheat or rye bread.

**For dinner** Introduce some extra chopped vegetables, such as fennel, celery, broccoli, or cabbage, at the same time as you add the peppers.

# Healthy soups

These soups are a great option for a quick dinner or lunch. They can all be kept chilled in the fridge for up to three days, so they are good options for making in bulk to save time on preparation. The gazpacho and mushroom soups can also be frozen for up to one month. All are complete meals that include protein, and all serve two.

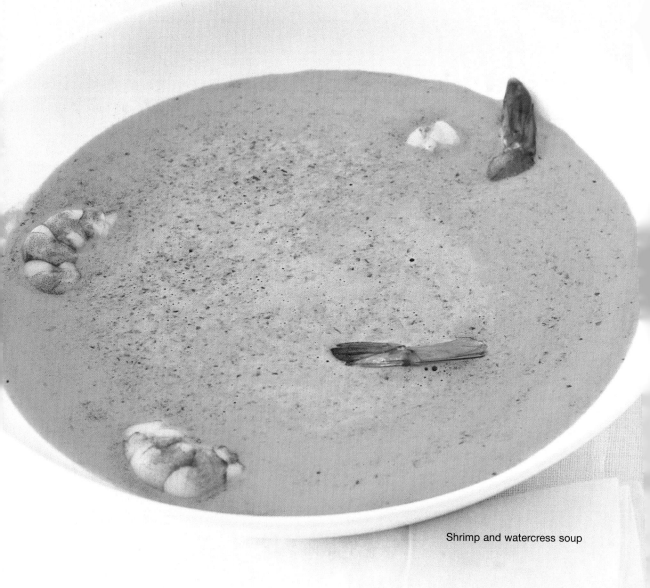

Shrimp and watercress soup

> ### SERVING IDEAS
>
> **For lunch** Serve with a piece of rye bread or a crusty whole-wheat roll.
>
> **For dinner** Add a few extra vegetables to the soup, such as corn or peas, to increase the complex-carbohydrate quotient.

## Shrimp and watercress soup

ready in **10** minutes

2 bunches watercress (approx. 5oz/150g), roughly shredded

Approx. 1½oz (45g) baby spinach leaves, coarsely chopped

3 large sprigs parsley

2 sprigs mint

2 cups (500ml) vegetable stock (*see p.149*)

Juice of ½ lemon

Freshly ground black pepper, to taste

¾ cup plain yogurt

1 egg

12–16 cooked shrimp

Mint or basil, to garnish

Put all the ingredients, except the shrimp and garnish, in a blender. Blend thoroughly to make a very fine mixture. Pour into a saucepan and heat gently until simmering. Although the egg will keep the yogurt from curdling, the soup should still not be boiled hard or simmered for too long.

Divide the shrimp between two bowls, cover with the soup, and serve garnished with the mint or basil.

## Mushroom and lentil soup

ready in **30** minutes

1¼ cups (300g) mushrooms, roughly chopped

½ cup (125g) chopped onion

2 tablespoons olive oil

1 bay leaf

3 sprigs fresh thyme or 1 teaspoon dried thyme

2 cups (500ml) vegetable stock (*see p.149*)

2 tablespoons tomato purée

Freshly ground black pepper, to taste

1 tablespoon soy sauce

1 approx. 13oz (400g) can lentils, drained and rinsed

2 tablespoons plain yogurt

Put the mushrooms and onion in a food processor and mix until the vegetables form a paste.

Heat the oil in a heavy saucepan over medium heat, add the mushroom and onion paste and the herbs. Cook for 5 minutes. Add the stock, tomato purée, and soy sauce. Bring to a boil, then lower the heat and simmer for 20 minutes. Remove the whole herbs from the pan, then stir in the lentils and season with black pepper to taste. Heat everything together for about 5 minutes. Divide the soup between two bowls, stir a tablespoon of yogurt into each, and serve.

## Very quick gazpacho

ready in **10** minutes

1 small red onion (approx. 5oz/150g), roughly chopped

1 pepper, any color, cored, seeded, and roughly chopped

½ cucumber (approx. 5oz/150g), roughly chopped

1 can (approx. 13oz/400g) tomatoes

1 tablespoon lemon juice

1 tablespoon olive oil

1 tablespoon tomato purée

1 cup (250ml) mixed vegetable juice

Large sprig parsley

2–3 sprigs basil

Freshly ground black pepper

3oz (90g) flaked cooked fish, chicken, or smoked mackerel (or ¼ cup chickpeas)

Finely chopped scallion, cucumber, and tomato, mixed, to garnish

Put all the ingredients, except the fish or chicken and the garnish mixture (but including the juice from the can of tomatoes), into a blender. Blend until smooth.

Divide the fish or chicken between two bowls and cover with the cold soup. Top with a tablespoon of the garnish mixture before serving.

# Chicken and cashew stir-fry

Stir-fries are a healthy option because they use little oil and the vegetables can be just lightly cooked so they retain their nutrients. Serves two.

**ready in 20 minutes**

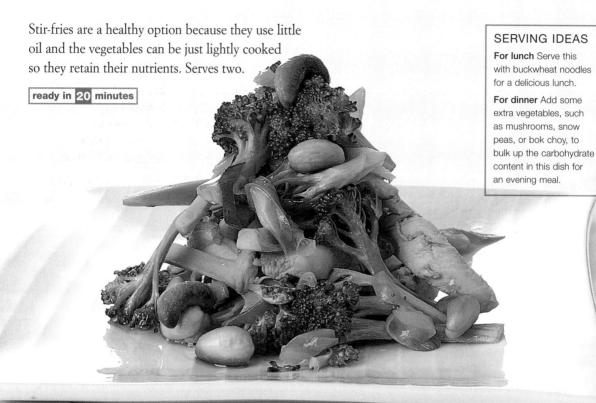

> **SERVING IDEAS**
>
> **For lunch** Serve this with buckwheat noodles for a delicious lunch.
>
> **For dinner** Add some extra vegetables, such as mushrooms, snow peas, or bok choy, to bulk up the carbohydrate content in this dish for an evening meal.

1 boneless, skinless chicken breast (approx. ¼lb/150g)

1 teaspoon five-spice powder (*see p.148*)

1 teaspoon tamarind paste, if available (*see p.149*)

1 tablespoon soy sauce

1 garlic clove, minced

Juice of ½ lemon

1 tablespoon white wine or water

¼ cup (60g) unsalted cashews

1 tablespoon olive oil

½ cup (125g) broccoli florets

2 scallions, trimmed and cut lengthways into 3in (7cm) strips

Cut the chicken into strips. Place the five-spice powder and tamarind paste (if it's available), soy sauce, garlic, lemon juice, and wine or water in a bowl and mix well together. Add the chicken strips and set aside to marinate for as much time as you have—about 30 minutes is preferable.

Heat a wok or frying pan over medium heat, add the cashews and dry-roast, turning often, until golden. Tip out of the pan onto a plate and set aside.

Pour the olive oil into the pan and heat gently. Lift the chicken strips from the marinade with a slotted spoon, add to the pan, and stir-fry for about 5 minutes. Add the marinade, broccoli, and scallions to the pan and continue cooking for another 5 minutes, adding a little more water if the contents begin to look a little dry. Finally, stir in the cashews and serve.

# Vegetable and bean soup

This recipe makes approximately eight servings. Any leftovers can be kept in the refrigerator for up to three days or frozen for up to one month.

**ready in 25 minutes**

2 tablespoons olive oil

2 onions (approx. 10oz/300g), chopped

2 garlic cloves, chopped

2 celery stalks, trimmed and finely sliced

3½oz (100g) green beans, trimmed and cut into 1⅛in (3cm) pieces

1 teaspoon ground coriander

1 can (approx. 13oz/400g) chopped tomatoes

3½ cups (1 liter) vegetable stock (*see p.149*)

½ cup (100g) shredded green cabbage

2 carrots (approx. 7oz/200g), grated

1 can (approx. 13oz /400g) cannellini beans

Grated Parmesan cheese to garnish

Heat the oil in a large, heavy saucepan over medium heat. Add the onions and cook gently for about 5 minutes, until the onions are softened.

Add the garlic, celery, green beans, and ground coriander to the pan, stir well, and cook for 5 minutes. Add the tomatoes and stock and simmer for an additional 5 minutes. Add the cabbage, carrots, and cannellini beans and simmer together for 5–10 minutes.

Sprinkle with a little grated Parmesan cheese and serve.

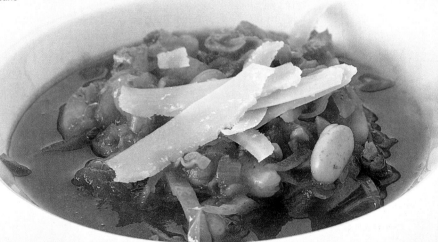

### SERVING IDEAS

**For lunch** This soup already contains everything you need for a warm lunch. Serve with a whole-wheat roll.

**For dinner** Add some extra celery, green beans, and cabbage if you wish, or serve with a side salad (*see pp.120–21*).

# Wraps and fillings

If you make a batch of the basic pancake wrap recipe, you can store the wraps in the refrigerator for one day or freeze them for up to one month. When freezing, separate them with plastic wrap or foil. To reheat them, add one at a time to a small frying pan. When the first side is hot, flip the pancake over. Each filling recipe serves two.

## Basic pancake wrap

ready in **20** minutes

½ cup (100g) buckwheat flour

1 large egg

1 cup (250ml) liquid (use ½ cup/125ml each milk and water, or all water)

Freshly ground black pepper, to taste

Put the flour into a large bowl. Make a well in the middle and break in the egg. Using a whisk, gradually add the liquid, whisking well, until the mixture has the consistency of thin cream. Depending on the size of the egg, you may need a little more or less fluid than the quantity specified. Add the black pepper to taste.

Wipe a little light-flavored oil with a paper towel over a flat frying pan or griddle and heat. When hot, pour an eighth of the mixture into the center of the pan, tilting the pan to spread the mixture. Cook for a minute or two until the pancake begins to bubble around the edge. Flip it over with a spatula and continue cooking for another minute or two.

When the pancake is cooked, turn it onto a plate lined with plastic wrap and continue making pancakes—the mixture should make eight. As you make them, continue to stack the pancakes on the plate, separated by plastic wrap.

## Wild mushroom and prosciutto wrap

ready in **15** minutes

2 tablespoons olive oil

8oz (250g) mixed wild mushrooms, sliced

6 sun-dried tomatoes in olive oil, cut in strips

Zest of ½ lemon

1 tablespoon chopped fresh parsley

Freshly ground black pepper, to taste

2 pancake wraps (*see left*)

2 handfuls mixed salad leaves

Walnut oil, to drizzle

2 slices prosciutto, cut into strips

1 tablespoon lemon juice

Heat the olive oil in a frying pan over medium heat, add the mushrooms, tomatoes, and lemon zest and cook for 10 minutes, or until the mushrooms are cooked. Stir in the parsley and black pepper.

Place each wrap on a plate, put a handful of salad leaves on each, and drizzle with walnut oil. Put half the mushroom mixture, a slice of prosciutto, and some lemon juice on each and roll them up to finish.

Wild mushroom and prosciutto wrap

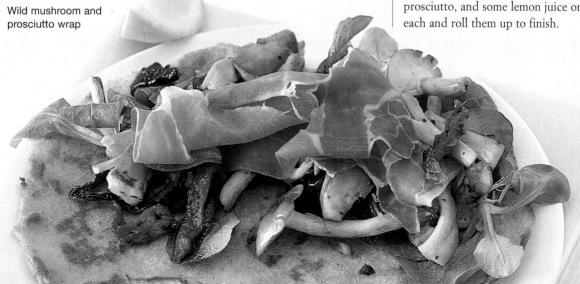

## Sesame, spinach, and poached egg wrap

ready in **10** minutes

1 heaping tablespoon sesame seeds

2 tablespoons olive oil

1 small onion, finely chopped

1 garlic clove, chopped

½lb (250g) fresh spinach, washed and coarsely shredded

1 tablespoon lemon juice

Freshly ground black pepper, to taste

2 eggs

2 pancake wraps (*see opposite*)

Heat a wok or frying pan over medium heat, put in the sesame seeds and dry-roast gently until golden. Set aside in a small bowl.

Heat the olive oil in the pan, add the onion and garlic, and cook until they start turning golden. Add the spinach leaves, lemon juice, and pepper. Stir-fry until the spinach is wilted, then set aside.

Break the eggs into a saucer and slide them into a pan of simmering water to which a dash of vinegar has been added. Poach the eggs until firm, then lift them from the pan with a slotted spoon and set aside to drain while you reheat or make the pancakes.

Put half the spinach mixture and one egg on half the pancake, sprinkle with half the sesame seeds, and fold the other half over. Leave in the pan for a few minutes for everything to heat together. Repeat with the second pancake.

## Asian-style squid wrap

ready in **20** minutes

½lb (250g) squid (cleaned weight), cleaned and cartilage removed

2½in (6cm) piece from the fat end of a lemon grass stalk, finely sliced

1½ tablespoons lime juice

1 tablespoon Thai fish sauce

½in (1cm) piece fresh ginger, peeled and grated

2 scallions, trimmed and sliced

½ orange, yellow, or red pepper, cored, seeded, and chopped

2 pancake wraps (*see opposite*)

Large handful of mixed salad leaves

Walnut or sesame oil, to drizzle

Few basil leaves

Few cilantro leaves

Slice the squid sacs into rings and roughly chop the tentacles. Drop them into a pan of boiling water and simmer for about one minute, or until the pieces are opaque and tender. Drain and set aside.

Place the lemongrass in a bowl with the lime juice, fish sauce, ginger, scallions, and pepper. Add the squid and mix everything well.

Lay the pancake wraps on a flat surface and divide the mixed salad leaves between them. Drizzle some oil over the leaves and top each wrap with half the squid mixture. Tear a few basil and cilantro leaves over each and roll them up.

Note: If you prefer, the squid may easily be replaced with tuna or cooked shrimp.

## Avocado and scallop wrap

ready in **10** minutes

1 ripe avocado, pitted, peeled, and cubed

8 ripe cherry tomatoes, quartered

1 tablespoon snipped chives

2 handfuls mixed salad leaves

1 tablespoon olive oil

4 scallops, halved horizontally

2 pancake wraps (*see opposite*)

**For the dressing:**

3 tablespoons olive oil

1 tablespoon lime juice

1 tablespoon chopped parsley

1 teaspoon Dijon mustard

Freshly ground black pepper, to taste

To make the dressing, place all the ingredients in a bowl and mix well.

Put the avocado, tomatoes, and chives in a bowl and cover with two-thirds of the dressing. Set aside. Heat the olive oil in a frying pan over medium heat and cook the scallops for 2 minutes on each side.

Lay both wraps on plates. Place a handful of salad leaves, the avocado mixture, and the remaining dressing on each and top with the scallops.

# Leeks in red pesto and tofu sauce

**LUNCH OR DINNER**

A delicious way of cooking leeks, this recipe works just as well with bulbs of fennel, which should be quartered or cut into thick slices before steaming. Serves two.

**ready in 20 minutes**

**SERVING IDEAS**

**For lunch** Serve with some rye bread and mixed leaves drizzled with a dressing *(see pp.114–15)*.

**For dinner** Add an extra leek to the recipe or try a mixture of both fennel and leek.

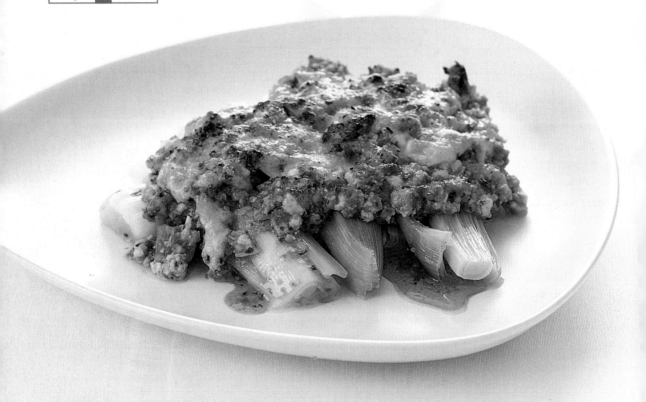

4 medium leeks

4 tablespoons red pesto *(see p.69)*

2½oz (75g) silken tofu

Juice of ½ lemon

½–¾ cup (125–150ml) vegetable stock *(see p.149)*

Freshly ground black pepper, to taste

Manchego cheese, finely grated

Trim and wash the leeks and slice each one in half vertically. Place in a steamer, or in a colander with a lid, over a saucepan of boiling water and steam for about 10–15 minutes, until soft.

Meanwhile, mix the red pesto, tofu, and lemon juice together in a bowl and add sufficient stock or vegetable juice to make a thick pouring sauce. Pour into a saucepan and bring to the simmering point. Add the black pepper.

When the leeks are cooked, put them in a heat-proof dish, cover with the sauce, and scatter the grated cheese on top. Place under the broiler for a couple of minutes until the cheese has browned on top, then serve.

# Cajun-style fish fry

**LUNCH** OR **DINNER**

The baby corn cobs can be replaced with the same weight of corn kernels, if you prefer. If you do not have onion powder, use a teaspoon of finely chopped onion instead. Serves two.

ready in **15** minutes

½lb (250g) firm white fish fillets, such as orange roughy, snapper, rockfish, cod, or haddock, cut into chunks

½ teaspoon each paprika, cinnamon, nutmeg, ginger, black pepper, and onion powder, mixed

¼ cup (60g) baby corn cobs, thickly sliced, or ¼ cup (60g) corn kernels

4oz (125g) sugar snap peas, trimmed

1 zucchini (approx. 4oz/125g), thickly sliced

2 tablespoons olive oil

Juice of ½ lemon

Chopped cilantro, to garnish

### SERVING IDEAS

**For lunch** Serve with buckwheat noodles and a mixed leaf salad.

**For dinner** Add some extra vegetables such as broccoli or cabbage.

Put the fish in a bowl, sprinkle with the mixed spices, and toss together well. Set aside to marinate.

Place the vegetables in a small pan, pour in water to just cover them, and bring to a boil. Simmer for about half a minute, then drain the vegetables.

Heat the olive oil in a wok or frying pan over medium-high heat, add the fish chunks, and stir-fry carefully for about 5 minutes, until cooked through and golden brown. Do not let the fish chunks fall to pieces. Lift them from the pan with a slotted spoon and set aside. Add the vegetables and lemon juice to the pan and stir-fry for 5 minutes or so, until the vegetables are hot. Carefully stir in the fish, scatter the cilantro over the top, and serve.

# Simple stir-fries

Stir-fries can be a great solution when you are in need of a quick, nutritious meal. They are also very versatile, so feel free to experiment with any vegetables you have in the refrigerator, rather than always sticking to those listed in the recipe. Each recipe serves two.

## Shrimp and sweet chili stir-fry

ready in **15** minutes

2 tablespoons olive oil

3 scallions, trimmed and finely sliced

¼lb (100g) snow peas, trimmed

½ red pepper, cored, seeded, and sliced

3½oz (100g) mushrooms, sliced

3½oz (100g) bean sprouts

¼ cup (75g) shredded Chinese cabbage

½lb (200g) cooked jumbo shrimp

**For the Sweet chili sauce:**

1 teaspoon honey

½ teaspoon chili powder

1 garlic clove, roughly chopped

½in (1cm) piece fresh ginger, peeled and grated

2 tablespoons cider vinegar

2 teaspoons Thai fish sauce

¼ cup (75g) vegetable stock (*see p.149*)

First make the sauce. Put all the ingredients in a bowl and mix well together. Add the shrimp and let stand while preparing the vegetables.

Heat the oil in a wok or frying pan over medium-high heat, add the scallions, and stir-fry for a minute.

Add the snow peas, pepper, and mushrooms, and stir-fry for 3–4 minutes until the ingredients are hot and the peas are beginning to wilt. Add the bean sprouts and cabbage, stirring to coat with the oil. Pour in the shrimp and sauce and simmer together for another 3–4 minutes, until everything is heated through. Serve immediately.

Shrimp and sweet chili stir-fry

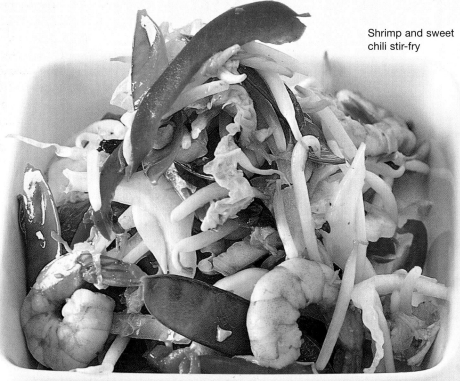

## Feta, tomato, and bean stir-fry

ready in **10** minutes

¼lb (150g) green beans, trimmed

2 tablespoons pine nuts

1 tablespoon olive oil

1 garlic clove, finely chopped

1 tablespoon lemon juice

1 heaped teaspoon Dijon mustard

6 cherry tomatoes, halved

4 sun-dried tomatoes in oil, drained and finely sliced

1oz (30g) black olives, pitted

½ can (13oz/400g) red kidney beans, drained and rinsed

1 tablespoon balsamic vinegar

2 large sprigs fresh thyme, finely chopped

Freshly ground black pepper, to taste

3½oz (100g) feta cheese, crumbled

Basil leaves, roughly torn, for garnishing

Cook the green beans in simmering water for one minute, drain, and set aside.

Heat a wok or frying pan over medium heat. Gently dry-roast the pine nuts for 2 minutes until light brown, stirring constantly. Remove from the pan and set aside.

Heat the oil in the wok. Add the green beans and garlic and cook for 1–2 minutes. Add the lemon juice and mustard, stirring to coat the beans. Mix in the tomatoes and stir until juice begins to run. Add the olives, red kidney beans, vinegar, thyme, and black pepper. When these are hot, stir in the pine nuts and cheese. Garnish with basil leaves and serve.

## Sesame ribbon stir-fry

ready in **20** minutes

1 sweet potato (approx. ¼lb/150g), peeled or two carrots (approx. ¼lb/150g), scrubbed and trimmed

1 zucchini (approx. ¼lb/150g), halved lengthways with seeds scraped out

3 tablespoons olive oil

3 scallions, trimmed and finely sliced lengthways

1 garlic clove, crushed

1 tablespoon lemon juice

1 tablespoon sesame seeds, to garnish

**For the egg ribbons:**

2 eggs

1 tablespoon water

Freshly ground black pepper, to taste

2 tablespoons chopped cilantro

1 tablespoon olive oil

**For the sauce:**

2 tablespoons soy sauce

1 tablespoon sesame oil

1 tablespoon cider vinegar

¼–½ teaspoon chili powder

½ teaspoon honey

1 tablespoon water

First make the egg ribbons. Put all the ingredients in a bowl and beat together lightly. Make a flat omelet (*see egg ribbons with cumin rice, p.139*). Roll up the omelet while it is warm and leave to cool while preparing the rest of the stir-fry.

To make the sauce, mix all the ingredients together in a bowl, then set aside.

Use a potato or vegetable peeler to peel the sweet potato or carrots and cut the zucchini into strips.

Heat the oil in a wok or frying pan over medium heat. Add the scallions and garlic and stir-fry for a minute. Add the sweet potato or carrot strips and stir-fry for about 2 minutes, then add the zucchini strips and lemon juice. Stir-fry for about 3 minutes until the vegetables are hot and wilting. Add the sauce and bring to the simmering point. Quickly slice the rolled-up omelet into ribbons.

Serve topped with the egg ribbons and garnished with the sesame seeds.

---

**SERVING IDEAS**

**For lunch** Serve any of these stir-fries with a portion of rice noodles for the perfect lunch.

**For dinner** Either add some extra vegetables to the stir-fry itself or pair with your choice of salad leaves.

# Seared tuna with beans and pasta

If you don't have any fresh tuna available, you can make this dish with canned tuna that is packed in spring water, rather than oil. Serves two.

**ready in 20 minutes**

3oz (90g) dried pasta (use buckwheat, corn, or whole-wheat)

2 teaspoons olive oil

¼lb (100g) green beans, trimmed and cut in half

½ red or orange pepper, cored, seeded, and sliced

1 fresh tuna steak (¼lb/100g)

2 tablespoons (30g) very finely sliced red onion

**For the dressing:**

4 tablespoons olive oil

2 tablespoons lemon juice

1 garlic clove, crushed

2 tablespoons chopped fresh parsley

Cook the pasta according to the instructions on the package. Drain into a colander and return to the empty pan. Drizzle with a teaspoon of the olive oil to prevent sticking and set aside.

Steam the beans and peppers over a pot of gently simmering water for about 5 minutes, or until cooked but still firm.

Brush the tuna with olive oil and sear in a pan or under the broiler, turning at least once, for 6–8 minutes, or until just cooked. Break the tuna into chunks.

To make the dressing, put all the ingredients in a bowl and mix well with a fork.

Put the pasta, beans, peppers, tuna chunks, and red onion in a large serving bowl, cover with the dressing, and toss to mix everything together well. (If you are using canned tuna, add it at this point.) Serve immediately.

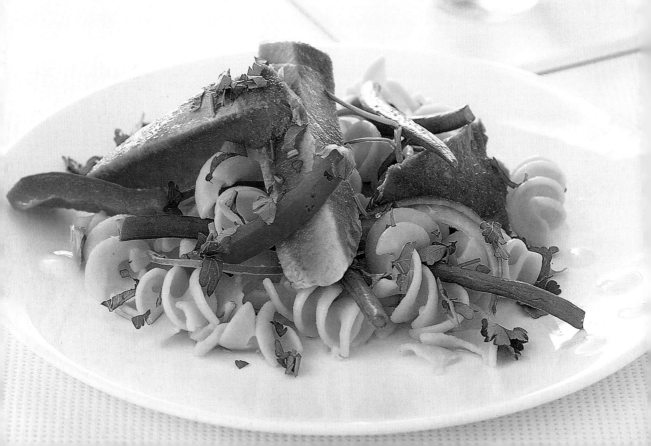

# Smoked chicken in sweet chili sauce

If you do not have smoked chicken, use grilled or broiled chicken instead—even leftover grilled chicken will do. Serves two.

**ready in 10 minutes**

### SERVING IDEAS

**For lunch** Serve with some brown rice or buckwheat noodles.

**For dinner** Add a handful of spinach, broccoli florets, or any other green vegetables at the same point as the sugar snap peas.

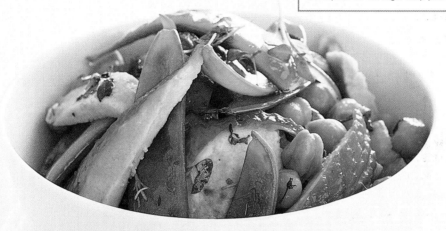

1 tablespoon olive oil

¼ cup (75g) sugar snap peas

¼ cup (60g) finely sliced onion

1 garlic clove, crushed

1 can (5oz/150g) chickpeas, drained and rinsed

3–4 sprigs thyme, chopped

¼ lb (100g) smoked chicken, cut into short strips

**For sweet chili sauce:**

1 heaping teaspoon chili paste

2 tablespoons orange juice

1 teaspoon lemon juice

1 small teaspoon honey, mixed with 3 tablespoons water

First, make the sweet chili sauce. Put all the ingredients in a bowl and whisk together with a fork.

Heat the oil in a wok or frying pan over medium heat, add the sugar snap peas and onion, and cook until the onion is soft. Add the garlic, chickpeas, and sauce and cook until the chickpeas are hot. Add the thyme and chicken and continue to cook, stirring, until the chicken is hot, then serve.

# Root vegetable and goat cheese salad

**LUNCH OR DINNER**

For this substantial salad, use celery root and carrots as the base vegetables, then add your favorites from among root vegetables, such as sweet potatoes, rutabagas, and parsnips. Serves two.

**ready in 10 minutes**

### SERVING IDEAS

**For lunch** Serve with a chunk of rye bread or a spoonful of couscous.

**For dinner** Increase the quantity of root vegetables and add another five cubes or so of goat cheese.

½lb (200g) root vegetables, coarsely grated

2 tablespoons olive oil

1 tablespoon black mustard seeds

1oz (30g) walnut pieces

2 tablespoons (25g) raisins

3½oz (100g) Manchego, mozzarella, or feta cheese, cubed

Sesame oil, to drizzle

1–2 tablespoons chopped fresh cilantro

Place the grated vegetables in a large bowl. Heat the oil in a small pan and, when hot, add the black mustard seeds. When the seeds start to pop, pour them over the vegetables. Stir in the walnuts, raisins, and cheese. Drizzle with sesame oil and sprinkle with the cilantro.

# Green and white salad

Since all the ingredients in this salad are quite delicately flavored, you can choose a tangy dressing to spice it up. Serves two.

ready in **10** minutes

3½oz (100g) cauliflower, broken into small florets

3½oz (100g) broccoli, broken into small florets

1 small carrot, grated

2½oz (75g) feta cheese, cut into chunks

2 tablespoons pumpkin seeds

2–3 tablespoons dressing (*choose from the dressings on pp.114–15*)

Put all the ingredients except the dressing in a salad bowl. Sprinkle with the dressing and toss everything together so that the vegetables are well coated, then serve.

## SERVING IDEAS

**For lunch** Serve with a few new potatoes drizzled with olive oil.

**For dinner** Add a few extra broccoli or cauliflower florets.

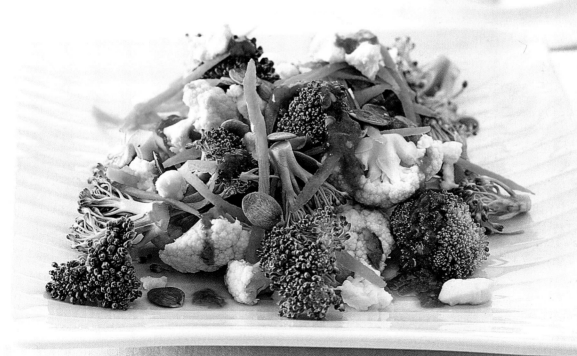

# Dressings

Many commercial dressings are laden with hidden "extras," such as saturated and trans fats, and sugar. Replace them with these dressings, which are delicious and quick, yet still diet-friendly They can be made in advance and kept in a sealed container in the refrigerator for up to five days. Each recipe serves two.

<table>
<tr><td>

**SERVING IDEAS**

**For lunch** Toss through any selection of mixed greens or salad vegetables, or mix into rice or couscous, to make a great accompaniment to any protein.

**For dinner** A plain salmon fillet with steamed green vegetables can be transformed by one of these dressings.

</td></tr>
</table>

## Coconut and lime dressing

ready in **5** minutes

2 tablespoons coconut milk

2 tablespoons lime juice

1 tablespoon plain yogurt

½ teaspoon Thai fish sauce (optional)

½ teaspoon Thai curry sauce

Combine all the ingredients in a bowl or screw-top jar, mix well and serve.

## Lemon and carrot juice dressing

ready in **5** minutes

¼ cup (60ml) carrot juice

3 tablespoons olive oil

1 tablespoon plain yogurt

1 tablespoon lemon juice

½ teaspoon red chili paste (or ¼ teaspoon cayenne pepper)

Freshly ground black pepper, to taste

Combine all the ingredients in a bowl or screw-top jar, mix well and serve.

Lime and soy dressing

Lemon and carrot juice dressing

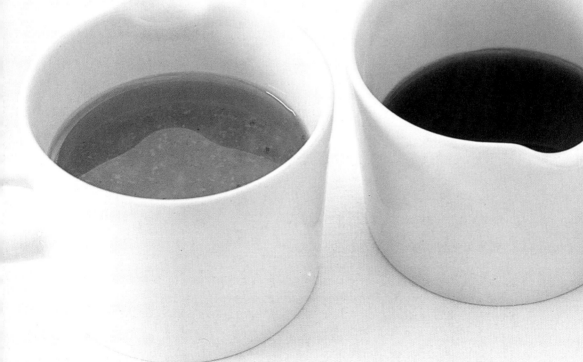

## Lime and soy dressing

ready in **5** minutes

2 tablespoons lime juice

2 tablespoons sesame oil

2 tablespoons avocado oil (or olive oil)

2 tablespoons olive oil

1 teaspoon soy sauce

1 garlic clove, crushed

Freshly ground black pepper, to taste

Combine all the ingredients in a bowl or screw-top jar, mix well and serve.

## Orange vinaigrette

ready in **5** minutes

6 tablespoons olive oil

2 tablespoons orange juice

1 tablespoon cider vinegar

½ teaspoon Dijon mustard

1 garlic clove, crushed and finely chopped

Freshly ground black pepper, to taste

Combine all the ingredients in a bowl or screw-top jar, mix well and serve.

## Sun-dried tomato dressing

ready in **5** minutes

4 sun-dried tomatoes in olive oil, drained and quartered

½ cup (125ml) olive oil

2 tablespoons lemon juice

1 tablespoon water

½ teaspoon anchovy paste

1 garlic clove, crushed

Freshly ground black pepper, to taste

Put all the ingredients in a blender and blend until smooth and ready to serve.

Sun-dried tomato dressing

Orange vinaigrette

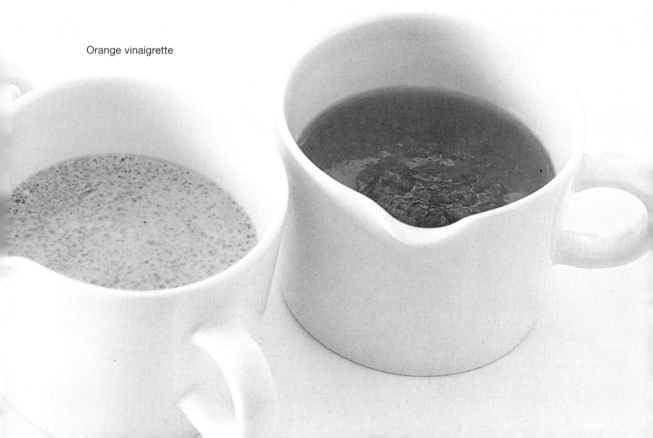

# Caesar salad

Here is a classic dish given the added-protein treatment. You could also reduce the quantities and omit the protein to create a side salad. Serves two.

**ready in 20 minutes**

3 tablespoons olive oil

1 garlic clove, finely chopped

2 thick slices rye bread (not pumpernickel), cubed

1 large head romaine lettuce, halved lengthways, rinsed, and dried

2 scallions, trimmed and finely sliced

2 tablespoons chopped fresh flat parsley

¼lb (150g) baked, broiled, or grilled chicken, smoked trout, or spicy chicken (*see pp.130–31*)

Parmesan cheese, finely sliced or grated

**For the dressing:**

2 tablespoons mayonnaise

1 tablespoon yogurt

1 tablespoon water

1 tablespoon lemon juice

1 tablespoon olive oil

1 garlic clove, crushed

1 teaspoon anchovy paste (if available) or a few anchovy fillets from a can or jar

Freshly ground black pepper, to taste

Preheat the oven to 350°F/180°C/gas mark 4.

Put the oil and garlic in a bowl and mix together. Add the cubes of rye bread and toss in the oil until well coated. Spread the cubes on a baking sheet and bake in the oven for about 15 minutes, turning them once or twice. When the cubes are evenly toasted, remove from the oven and cool on an absorbent paper towel.

To make the dressing, put all the ingredients (except for the anchovy fillets, if you are using them), into a screw-top jar and shake well to mix.

Coarsely slice the lettuce halves and divide them between two large individual salad bowls. Scatter half the scallions and parsley over each. Top each bowl with half the rye croutons, chicken or trout, cheese (and anchovy fillets, if you are using them). Spoon 2–3 tablespoons of the dressing over each bowl and toss well before serving.

Note: Any dressing left over may be stored in a screw-top jar in the refrigerator for up to five days.

> **SERVING IDEAS**
>
> **For lunch** Add a few chopped new potatoes to the salad.
>
> **For dinner** Increase the amount of lettuce rather than adding some starchy carbohydrate as you would at lunch.

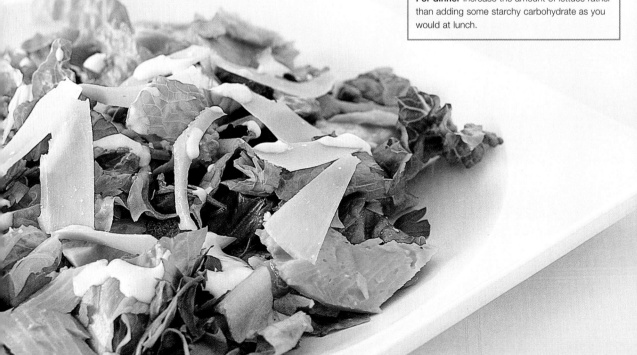

# Squash and feta rosti

This rosti is a great vegetarian option. It tastes just as good cold, so make a little extra and save some for the next morning's snack. Serves two.

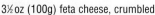

ready in **20** minutes

2 tablespoons olive oil

1 onion (approx. 3½ oz/100g), finely chopped

½ teaspoon caraway seeds

1in (2.5cm) piece fresh ginger, peeled and grated

11oz (325g) firm squash, such as butternut, peeled, seeded, and coarsely grated

3½ oz (100g) feta cheese, crumbled

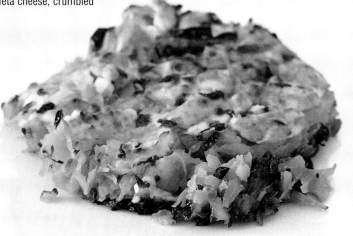

Heat the oil in a small nonstick frying pan over medium-high heat, add the onion and caraway seeds, and cook until the onion is softened and golden. Add the ginger and mix well. Mix in the grated squash and stir-fry gently for 3–4 minutes to soften the squash and combine the ingredients.

Cover with the crumbled feta and mix well. Pat down the mixture in the pan and draw it in from the sides to make a cake. Leave over medium-high heat for about 5 minutes to firm and brown the base.

Put the pan under the broiler for an additional 5 minutes to brown the top. Cut in half and serve.

## SERVING IDEAS

**For lunch** Serve with a piece of toasted rye or whole-grain bread.

**For dinner** The tomato and onion niçoise and the ratatouille (see pp.96–97 for recipes) make perfect moist side dish options for this crunchy rosti. Add some extra feta to increase the protein amount too.

# Asian fish cakes

These are so delicious you may not have leftovers, but if you do, mash them with a little salsa to make a great snack topping for crackers. Serves two.

**ready in 20 minutes**

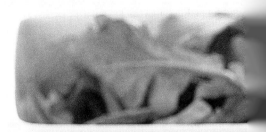

½lb (200g) white fish fillets, cut into chunks

4 scallions, trimmed and chopped

1 teaspoon grated fresh ginger

1 teaspoon green curry paste

2 teaspoons Thai fish sauce

1 egg

2 tablespoons chopped cilantro or parsley

2 tablespoons flour (gluten-free flour, rice flour, or cornstarch)

Zest of 1 lime

1 tablespoon lime juice

Freshly ground black pepper, to taste

### SERVING IDEAS

**For lunch** Serve the fish cakes with red or green salsa (*see pp.94–95*), new potatoes, and steamed vegetables or a green salad.

**For dinner** Try the cakes with the fennel and carrot side salad, or another from pp.120–21.

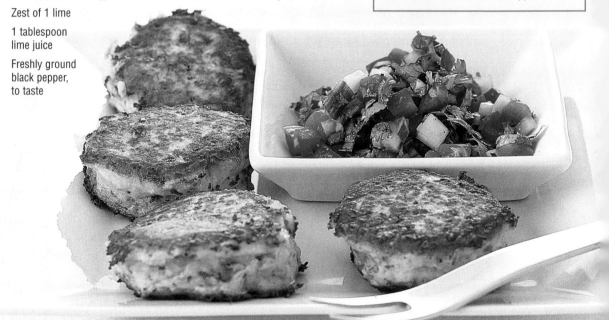

Place the fish chunks, scallions, ginger, curry paste, fish sauce, egg, and herbs in a food processor and blend until the mixture is fairly smooth, but still has some texture.

Scrape the mixture into a bowl. Add the flour, lime zest and juice, and black pepper, and stir gently to mix it all together. Divide the mixture into eight portions and, with lightly-floured hands, form each portion into a ball. The fish cakes may be steamed or shallow-fried.

To steam them: Place them in a steamer over simmering water, cover, and steam for 10 minutes.

To fry them: Slightly flatten each ball, then gently heat 3–4 tablespoons of olive oil in a shallow frying pan over medium heat, add the fish cakes, and cook gently for 5–8 minutes, turning them at intervals, until they are golden brown and cooked through.

Serve four fish cakes per portion.

# Sprouted seed salad

**LUNCH** OR **DINNER**

There is an enormous choice of sprouts available in supermarkets and particularly health-food stores. They are incredibly nutritious and are packed with antioxidants, vitamins, minerals, and amino acids. You could even grow your own sprouted seeds in only a few days. Serves two.

ready in **10** minutes

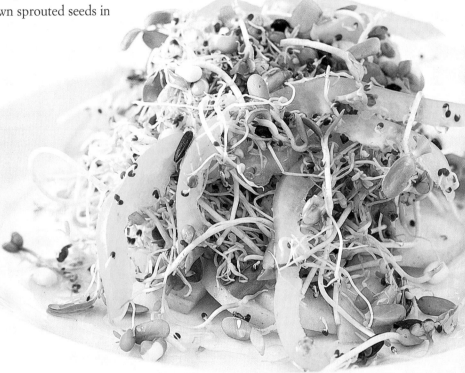

8oz (250g) mixed sprouted seeds and beans

1 large crisp apple, cored and sliced

1 yellow pepper, cored, seeded, and cut into strips

4 tablespoons chopped mixed fresh herbs (choose from parsley, cilantro, chives, dill, fennel, oregano, mint, and basil)

½ cup (125ml) dressing (*see pp.114–15*)

Put all the ingredients in a large salad bowl. Toss gently to mix everything together well.

## SERVING IDEAS

**For lunch** Add a small baked potato or a portion of brown rice.

**For dinner** Mix in some extra yellow pepper, or any other salad vegetables you may have available.

# Side salads

These fresh and nutritious salads are simple to make. Try them with the dressings on pp.114–15, then serve with the protein of your choice. Whether added to some grilled fish, or yesterday's leftover chicken, these salads will liven up any meal. Each recipe serves two.

## Avocado and watercress salad

| ready in | 5 | minutes |

2oz (60g) watercress, coarsely torn

Small handful arugula, coarsely torn

12 cherry tomatoes, halved

1 avocado, peeled, pitted, and cut into chunks

4 white mushroom caps, sliced

2–3 tablespoons dressing of your choice (*see pp.114–15*)

Mix the watercress and arugula in the bottom of a salad bowl, and pile the tomatoes, avocado, and mushrooms into the middle.

Drizzle the dressing over the top, being sure to cover the avocado chunks well to preserve their pretty green color. If you prefer, use a drizzle of walnut or olive oil instead of the dressing.

## Red and white cabbage salad

| ready in | 10 | minutes |

2 heaping teaspoons caraway seeds

4oz (125g) white cabbage, grated

2½oz (75g) red cabbage, grated

2–3 tablespoons dressing of your choice (*see pp.114–15*)

Put the caraway seeds in a heavy-bottomed pan and dry-roast them over a moderate heat for about 5 minutes, tossing occasionally.

Put both grated cabbages into a bowl, mix them together, then drizzle with the dressing. Mix everything together gently, and watch the red cabbage make pink trails through the salad. Top with the roasted caraway seeds and serve.

## Fennel and carrot salad

| ready in | 10 | minutes |

1 bulb fennel (approx. ¼lb/125g), trimmed with feathery fronds set aside

2 carrots (approx. 4oz/125g), coarsely grated

Juice of 1 lemon

2 teaspoons olive oil

2 teaspoons poppy seeds

Cut the fennel bulb in half lengthways and finely slice across each half. Put the fennel slices in a salad bowl and add the grated carrot and lemon juice.

Heat the olive oil in a small heavy-bottomed pan over a moderate heat for a couple of minutes, then add the poppy seeds. Once the seeds start to pop, pour them and the oil over the salad and toss it well. Serve the salad garnished with a few of the fennel fronds.

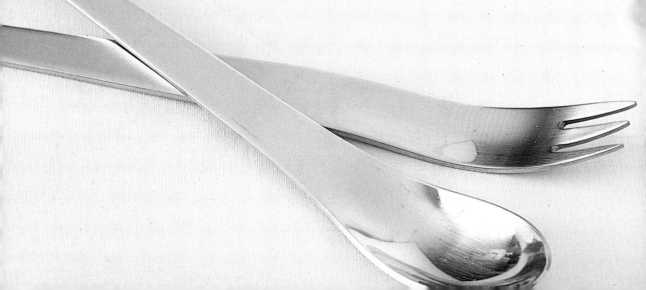

# High C salad

| ready in | 5 | minutes |

2 medium tomatoes, sliced

½ cucumber, halved lengthways and sliced

1 kiwi, peeled, halved lengthways, and sliced

2 tablespoons olive oil

2 tablespoons lemon juice

Freshly ground black pepper, to taste

Fresh basil, to garnish

Place all the ingredients, except the basil, in a salad bowl. Use a fork and spoon to toss the ingredients gently but thoroughly together. Garnish with shredded basil leaves.

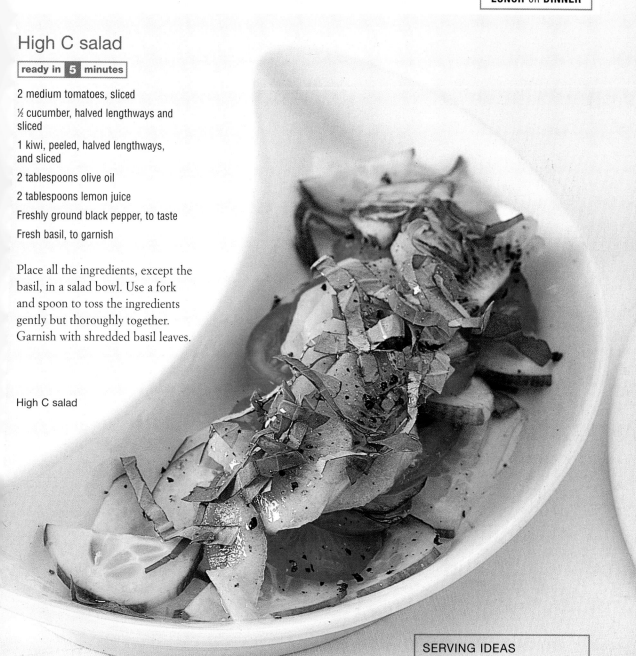

High C salad

## SERVING IDEAS

**For lunch** Try one of these salads with some grilled fish or chicken and a small baked potato for a perfect lunch.

**For dinner** Avoid the potatoes if you are eating after 7pm, and try one of these salads with a spicy chicken recipe from pp.130–31.

# Coconut and cilantro fish with couscous

**LUNCH OR DINNER**

Orange roughy is light and delicately flavored, but cod or monkfish fillets could be easily used instead, if that is what you have available. Serves two.

**ready in** 15 **minutes**

> ### SERVING IDEAS
>
> **For lunch** Serve with chopped cherry tomatoes and cucumber added to the couscous.
>
> **For dinner** Omit the couscous and in its place serve one of the side salads from pp.120–21.

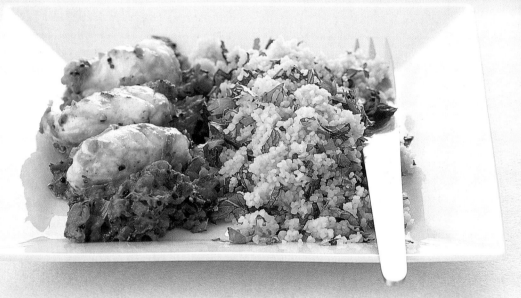

2 fillets (approx. ½–¾ lb/300g) orange roughy

Juice of 1 lime

Freshly ground black pepper, to taste

1 tablespoon olive oil

1 heaped teaspoon mustard seeds

2 small dried red chilies

1 garlic clove, finely chopped

1 small onion, finely sliced

2 tomatoes, chopped

½ cup (125ml) coconut milk

1 teaspoon ground coriander

2 tablespoons water

1 tablespoon chopped cilantro

### For the couscous:

½ cup (125g) couscous

¾ cup (175ml) lightly salted boiling water

2 teaspoons olive oil

1 tablespoon each chopped fresh parsley and cilantro

Preheat the oven to 275°F/140°C/gas mark 1. Cut each fillet into 3 pieces. Sprinkle with half the lime and some black pepper and set aside.

Put the couscous in an oven-proof bowl with the boiling water. Stir with a fork until the water is absorbed. Stir in the olive oil. Cover with foil and keep warm in the oven.

Heat the remaining olive oil over medium-high heat in a wok or frying pan, add the mustard seeds and chilies, and cook for 2 minutes. Add the garlic and onion and cook until the onion begins to color. Mix in the tomatoes, coconut, ground coriander seeds, remaining lime juice, and water. Stir-fry for 1–2 minutes. Add the fish and any juice and spoon the sauce over it. Cook very gently for about 5–6 minutes, until the fish is opaque. Serve the fish topped with the cilantro. Remove the couscous from the oven, stir in the herbs, add to the plates, and serve.

# Chicken in summer herbs with mixed bean salad

**LUNCH OR DINNER**

This mixed bean salad makes a substantial side dish, perfect for either lunch or dinner. Substitute thyme for rosemary for a different twist. Serves two.

**ready in 20 minutes**

1 tablespoon olive oil

1lb (250–300g) boneless, skinless chicken breast, cut into thick strips

1 garlic clove, chopped

8 scallions, trimmed and chopped

2 generous tablespoons chopped mixed fresh herbs (such as parsley, thyme, sage, chives, marjoram, basil, and tarragon)

2 tablespoons lemon juice

Freshly ground black pepper, to taste

**For the mixed bean salad:**

1 can (approx. 8oz/250g) mixed beans, drained and rinsed

4 sprigs fresh thyme (or 1 teaspoon dried)

½ cup (125ml) hot vegetable stock (*see p.149*)

1 tablespoon chopped fresh parsley

1 tablespoon olive oil

Juice of ½ lemon

Heat the oil over medium-high heat in a frying pan with a lid. Add the chicken strips and brown lightly on all sides, turning frequently to keep them from sticking to the pan. Reduce the heat, toss in the scallions, mixed herbs, lemon juice, and pepper, and cover the pan. Cook gently for about 10 minutes, stirring occasionally, until the chicken is cooked through but still moist.

Make the bean salad while the chicken is cooking. First, put the beans in a saucepan with the stock and thyme. Simmer uncovered until the stock is absorbed, around 5 minutes. Pick out the fresh thyme and serve with the parsley, olive oil, and lemon juice mixed in.

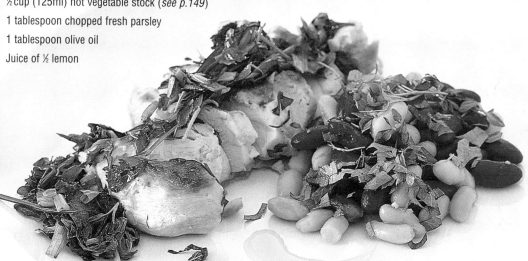

**SERVING IDEAS**

**For lunch** Add some rice or chopped new potatoes.

**For dinner** Serve the dish as it is but add a salad of mixed green leaves. For a lighter option, substitute the ratatouille (*see p.96*) for the mixed bean salad.

# Simple salmon

Salmon fillets have firm flesh with a fine texture and are bone-free. They work well with a wide variety of flavorful ingredients, as in these four recipes, which can be served hot or cold. Marinate the salmon fillets in foil packets for 15–20 minutes if time allows, so that the flavors of the ingredients are well absorbed. If you prefer, experiment with other firm fish as well, such as cod, tuna, or monkfish. Each recipe serves two.

### SERVING IDEAS

**For lunch** Any of these recipes would work well with steamed vegetables and new potatoes.

**For dinner** A peppery green salad of arugula and watercress makes an ideal simple accompaniment.

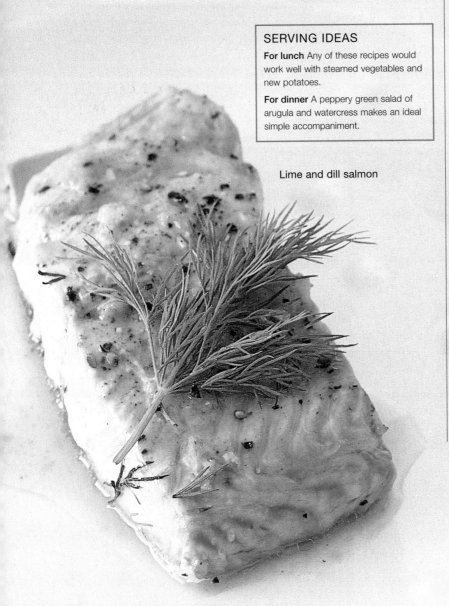

Lime and dill salmon

## Lime and dill salmon

ready in **20** minutes

2 salmon fillets (approx. ¼ lb/150g each), skin on

2 tablespoons lime juice

2 teaspoons grated fresh ginger

½ teaspoon anchovy paste (or 1 anchovy fillet in oil, drained and crushed)

6 large sprigs fresh dill

Freshly ground black pepper, to taste

Place each fillet, skin side down, on a square of aluminum foil large enough to fold over into a packet.

Put the lime juice, ginger, and anchovy paste or crushed anchovy fillet in a bowl, mix together well, and pour half the mixture over each fillet. Top each fillet with 2 sprigs of dill and a few twists of black pepper. Fold the foil loosely into packets and set aside for the fish to absorb the flavors while you prepare the rest of the meal.

A few minutes before you wish to cook the fish, preheat the oven to 300°F/150°C/gas mark 2. Cook the fish for 10–15 minutes until it is cooked through but still moist. Serve sprinkled with the juices from the packets and garnished with the remaining dill.

## Coconut and cilantro salmon

ready in **20** minutes

2 salmon fillets (approx. ¼ lb/150g each), skin on

⅛ cup (1½ tablespoons) coconut milk

2 tablespoons lemon juice

Freshly ground black pepper, to taste

6 large sprigs fresh cilantro

Place each fillet, skin side down, on a square of aluminum foil large enough to fold over into a packet.

Pour the coconut milk and half of lemon juice over each fillet, and sprinkle with pepper. Top each fillet with 2 sprigs of cilantro. Fold the foil loosely into packets and set aside for the fish to absorb the flavors while you prepare the rest of the meal.

A few minutes before you are ready to cook the fish, preheat the oven to 300°F/150°C/gas mark 2. Bake the fish for 10–15 minutes, until it is cooked through but still moist. Serve with the juices from the packets and the remaining lemon juice. Garnish with cilantro.

## Fennel and grapefruit salmon

ready in **20** minutes

2 salmon fillets (approx. ¼ lb/150g each), skin on

2 tablespoons grapefruit juice

½ teaspoon anchovy paste (or 1 anchovy fillet in oil, drained and crushed)

6 sprigs fresh fennel fronds

Freshly ground black pepper, to taste

Place each fillet, skin side down, on a square of aluminum foil large enough to fold over into a packet.

Place the grapefruit juice and anchovy paste or crushed anchovy fillet in a bowl, whisk together with a fork, and spoon half the mixture over each fillet. Top with 2 sprigs of fennel and a good grind of black pepper. Fold the foil loosely into packets and leave to stand while you prepare the rest of the meal.

A few minutes before you are ready to cook the fish, preheat the oven to 300°F/150°C/gas mark 2. Cook the fish for 10–15 minutes, until it is cooked through but still moist. Serve sprinkled with the juices from the packets and garnished with the remaining fennel sprigs.

## Soy and scallion salmon

ready in **20** minutes

2 salmon fillets (approx. ¼ lb/150g each), skin on

2 tablespoons orange juice

1 tablespoon soy sauce

2 scallions, trimmed and very finely sliced

6 sprigs fresh thyme

Place each fillet, skin side down, on a square of aluminum foil large enough to fold into a packet.

Put the orange juice and soy sauce in a small bowl and whisk together. Scatter the scallion slices evenly over the two fillets. Cover with the juice mixture and top each fillet with 2 thyme sprigs. Fold the foil loosely into a packet and leave to stand while you prepare the rest of the meal.

A few minutes before you wish to cook the fish, preheat the oven to 300°F/150°C/gas mark 2. Cook the fish for 10–15 minutes until it is cooked through but still moist. Serve sprinkled with the juices from the packets and garnished with the remaining thyme.

# Quick marinades

Marinades add flavor to meat and fish and help tenderize the portions before they are quickly seared on a grill pan or under the broiler. Just 15 or 20 minutes of marinating while the rest of a meal is prepared works wonders with many cuts of meat, poultry, fish, and even tofu.

## Chili, lime, and garlic marinade

ready in **5** minutes

1 tablespoon olive oil

2 garlic cloves, crushed

½ teaspoon chili paste

¼ teaspoon cayenne pepper

1 teaspoon paprika

Zest and juice of 1 lime

Combine all the ingredients in a bowl, add the chicken, meat, or fish, and stir or rub well to cover. Will keep in the fridge for at least a week.

## Horseradish and lime marinade

ready in **5** minutes

1 tablespoon prepared horseradish or horseradish sauce (*see p.148*)

1 tablespoon lime juice

½–1 tablespoon plain yogurt

1 tablespoon olive oil

Freshly ground black pepper, to taste

Put all the ingredients in a bowl and mix them well together. Pour over fish, poultry, or meat. Will keep in the fridge for about 3 days.

## Sesame oil and grainy mustard marinade

ready in **5** minutes

2 tablespoons sesame oil

1 tablespoon wholegrain mustard

1 tablespoon lemon juice

1 tablespoon orange juice

Freshly ground black pepper, to taste

Put all the ingredients in a bowl and mix well together. Rub into the fish or meat. The marinade will keep for 2–3 days in a screw-top jar in the refrigerator.

Sesame oil and grainy mustard

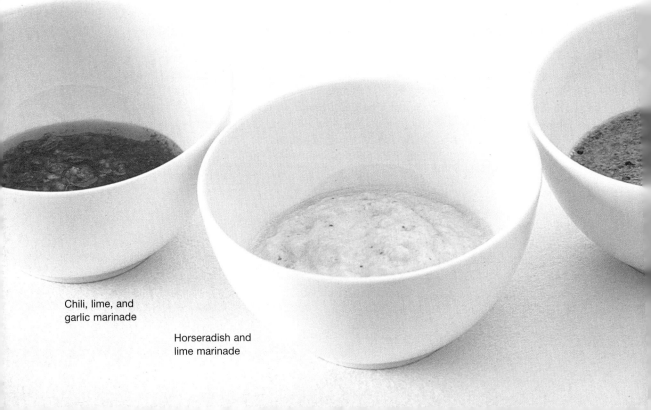

Chili, lime, and garlic marinade

Horseradish and lime marinade

## Tamarind and five-spice marinade

ready in **5** minutes

2 scallions, trimmed and cut into 2 or 3 pieces

2 tablespoons soy sauce

1 heaping teaspoon tamarind paste (*see p.149*)

1 small teaspoon honey

1 garlic clove, crushed

1 tablespoon five-spice powder (*see p.148*)

1 tablespoon cider vinegar

3½fl oz (100ml) water

Put all the ingredients in a heavy-bottomed saucepan, bring to a boil, for 2 minutes. The marinade may be used immediately, or cooled, poured into a screw-top jar, and stored in the refrigerator for 2–3 days.

## Yogurt and ginger marinade

ready in **5** minutes

3 tablespoons plain yogurt

1 heaping teaspoon grated fresh ginger

½ teaspoon turmeric

1 garlic clove, chopped

Freshly ground black pepper, to taste

Put all the ingredients in a bowl and mix them well together. Not only does the turmeric have a lovely subtle flavor—it also adds a wonderful color to meat or fish marinated in the mixture. Will keep in the fridge for about 3 days.

### SERVING IDEAS

**For lunch** Choose your favorite marinade, add it to your choice of protein, and serve it with new potatoes and a green salad.

**For dinner** The heat in the chili, lime, and garlic marinade goes well with fish or chicken and the fresh and tangy high C salad (*see p.121*).

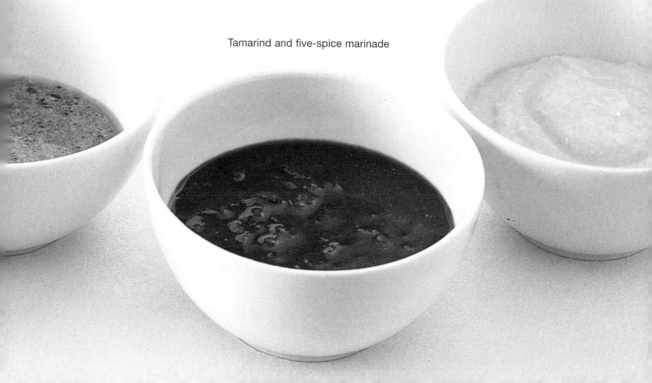

Yogurt and ginger marinade

Tamarind and five-spice marinade

# Cinnamon-seared tuna

Tuna is a fantastic protein option. It is a versatile, lean, and succulent fish, and, in this dish, it looks stunning enough for a dinner party. Serves two.

**ready in 20 minutes**

1 heaping teaspoon ground cinnamon

1 teaspoon ground ginger

1 teaspoon chili powder

2 tuna steaks (approx. ¼ lb/150g)

2 tablespoons olive oil

Put the cinnamon, ginger, and chili powder in a small bowl and stir well to mix. Rub each steak well on both sides first with the olive oil and then with the spice mixture. Set aside for 10–15 minutes so that the tuna absorbs the flavor of the spice mixture.

Heat a grill pan over high heat, put the tuna steaks in, and sear for 3–4 minutes on each side. Alternatively, heat the broiler to high and sear the tuna steaks, again for 3–4 minutes on each side. Don't overcook the fish. It should be only just cooked and still juicy as you serve it.

## SERVING IDEAS

**For lunch** Spiced rice (*see p.133*) will go very well with this tuna.

**For dinner** Serve with a large spoonful of the pea, ginger, and tapenade spread (*see p.66*) or some mixed leaves drizzled with your choice of dressing from pp.114–15.

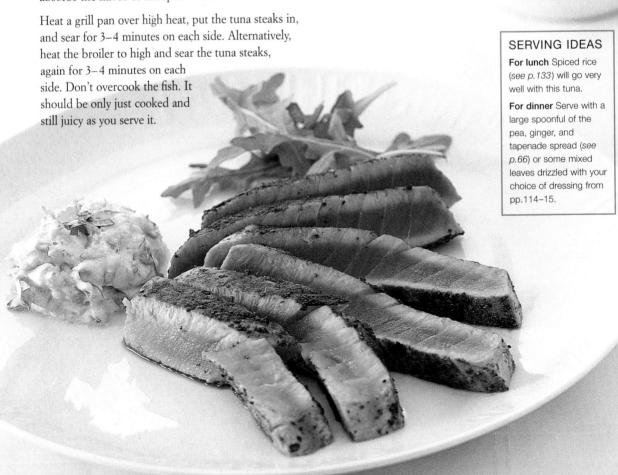

# Baked spinach scramble

Great for lunch or dinner, this dish also makes a delicious weekend breakfast—a new take on eggs florentine. Serves two.

| ready in **20** minutes |

2 tablespoons olive oil, plus extra for drizzling

2 slices whole-grain or rye bread, pulsed into fine crumbs in a food processor

½ teaspoon nutmeg

1lb (500g) spinach, washed and drained

Juice of 1 lemon

Juice of 1 orange

½ teaspoon cinnamon

Freshly ground black pepper, to taste

3 large eggs

2oz (60g) feta cheese, crumbled

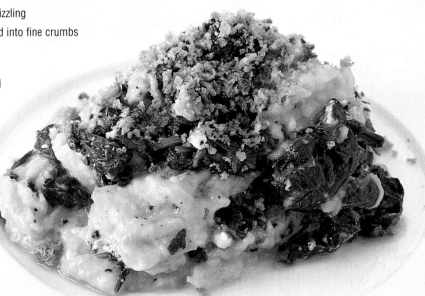

Heat 1 tablespoon of the oil over medium heat in a small pan, add the crumbs and nutmeg, and stir-fry until crisp. Tip the crumbs out of the pan onto a paper towel to drain and set aside.

Lightly cook the spinach. Either steam it for a couple of minutes until the leaves have wilted, or put the wet leaves into a large pan and cook very gently, turning frequently, until wilted. Drain the spinach and chop coarsely with scissors.

Heat the remaining oil in a heavy-bottomed pan over medium-low heat, then add the spinach, juices, cinnamon, and black pepper, and stir everything together. Break in the eggs and stir well over gentle heat to break them up, until curds form. Quickly stir in the feta.

Turn the egg mixture into a shallow oven-proof dish, and top with the toasted bread crumbs and a drizzle of olive oil. Brown under a medium-high broiler for 2–3 minutes, then serve.

### SERVING IDEAS

**For lunch** A slice of toasted and buttered soda bread goes well with this dish.

**For dinner** Increase the quantity of spinach in this dish or add some kale to the mixture.

# Spicy chicken

Chicken breasts are a great source of lean protein. These ideas give a tasty kick to a regular dish and are great for grilling. To grind the spices, you can use a traditional spice grinder, a coffee grinder, or a mortar and pestle. Each recipe serves two.

## Cajun-spiced chicken

ready in **15** minutes

2 boneless, skinless, chicken breasts (approx. 10oz/300g)

1 teaspoon olive oil

1 teaspoon lemon juice

**For the Cajun spice mix:**

½ teaspoon caraway seeds

½ teaspoon cumin seeds

1 teaspoon paprika

1 teaspoon cayenne or chili pepper

½ teaspoon freshly ground black pepper

1 teaspoon dried oregano

First, prepare the spice mix. Grind the caraway and cumin seeds and mix with the other herbs and spices.

Rub the chicken breasts with a little olive oil and lemon juice, then coat them with the spice mix.

Put the chicken breasts in a grill pan and cook under the broiler, or over medium heat on top of the stove, for about 6 minutes on each side, until cooked through but still juicy.

Slice the chicken breasts lengthways into four, then serve.

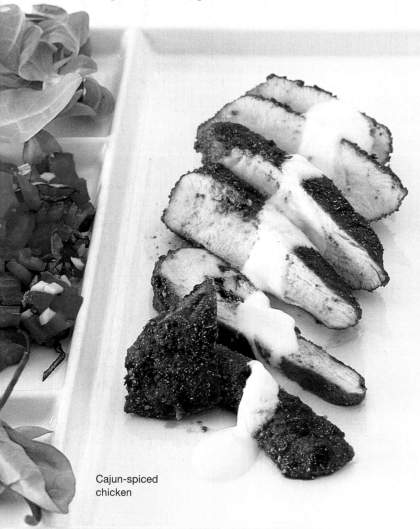

Cajun-spiced chicken

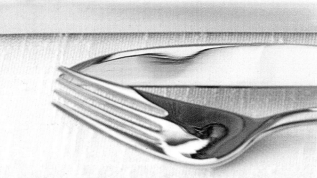

# Middle-eastern spicy chicken

ready in **15** minutes

2 boneless, skinless, chicken breasts (approx. 10oz/300g)

1 teaspoon olive oil

1 teaspoon lemon juice

1 teaspoon sesame oil

**For the Middle-eastern spice mix:**

6 teaspoons sesame seeds

3 teaspoons coriander seeds

3 teaspoons cumin seeds

Freshly ground black pepper, to taste

To dry-roast coriander seeds, put them in a heavy-bottomed pan over medium heat for 5–6 minutes, tossing occasionally to brown all sides and to prevent burning.

Put in a grinder, add the other spices, and grind to a powder.

Rub the chicken breasts with a little olive oil and lemon juice, then coat them with the spice mix.

Put the chicken breasts in a grill pan and cook under the broiler, or over medium heat on top of the stove, for about 6 minutes on each side, until cooked through but still juicy.

Slice the chicken breasts lengthways into four. Drizzle with a little sesame oil and serve.

# Garam masala spicy chicken

ready in **15** minutes

2 boneless, skinless, chicken breasts (approx. 10oz/300g)

1 teaspoon olive oil

1 teaspoon lemon juice

**For the garam masala spice mix:**

1 tablespoon cardamom pods

2in (5cm) cinnamon stick

1 teaspoon cumin seeds

1 teaspoon cloves

¼ of a nutmeg

Grind all the spices together. Rub the chicken breasts with a little olive oil and lemon juice, then coat them with the spice mix.

Put the chicken breasts in a grill pan and cook under the broiler, or over medium heat on top of the stove, for about 6 minutes on each side, until cooked through but still juicy.

Slice the chicken breasts lengthways into four and serve.

# Indian spicy chicken

ready in **15** minutes

2 boneless, skinless, chicken breasts (approx. 10oz/300g)

1 teaspoon olive oil

1 teaspoon lemon juice

**For the Indian spice mix:**

1 tablespoon coriander seeds, dry-roasted

½ teaspoon chili powder

½ teaspoon turmeric

Grind the coriander seeds (see Middle-eastern recipe for how to roast these) and mix with the chili and turmeric.

Rub the chicken breasts with a little olive oil and lemon juice, then coat them with the spice mix.

Put the chicken breasts in a grill pan and cook under the broiler, or over medium heat on top of the stove, for about 6 minutes on each side, until cooked through but still juicy.

Slice the chicken breasts lengthways into four. Drizzle with a little olive oil and serve.

---

**SERVING IDEAS**

**For lunch** Any of these would work well with red or green salsa (see p.94) or with plain yogurt and a spoonful of rice.

**For dinner** Serve with salad greens, steamed vegetables, or one of the side dishes on pp.96–97.

# Slow-burn side dishes

These four dishes are called slow-burning due to their low GI rating, which means they provide steady energy and fill you up for quite a while and don't trigger as much insulin as most high-carbohydrate side dishes. The three non-rice recipes also make great spreads for snacks if put in a blender. Each recipe serves two.

## Split yellow peas with scallions

**ready in 30 minutes**

½ cup (100g) split yellow peas (or split mung beans or split red lentils)

1 cup (250ml) water

¼ teaspoon turmeric

1 tablespoon olive oil

1 tablespoon lemon juice

1 scallion, trimmed and finely chopped

Freshly ground black pepper, to taste

Put the peas, water, and turmeric in a saucepan. Bring to a boil, cover the pan, reduce the heat, and simmer gently for 25 minutes until the peas are soft and the water has been absorbed. Add the olive oil, lemon juice, scallion, and black pepper. Stir well to combine the flavors before serving.

### SERVING IDEAS

**For lunch** Try a Mexican-style wrap (*see p.104*) of refried beans, guacamole or pea, ginger, and tapenade spread (*see p.66*), and some arugula leaves.

**For dinner** These can liven up a simple poached chicken or omelet, and work well with recipes such as squash and feta rosti (*see p.117*).

## Lima beans Italian-style

**ready in 20 minutes**

1 bag (approx. 10oz/275g) frozen lima beans, thawed

½ cup (125ml) vegetable stock (*see p.149*)

1 tablespoon olive oil

1 garlic clove, finely chopped

1 heaping tablespoon tomato purée

Freshly ground black pepper, to taste

1 tablespoon chopped fresh parsley, to garnish

Put the lima beans in a heavy-bottomed saucepan and add the hot stock. Bring to a boil and simmer gently to thoroughly heat the beans .

In a separate pan, heat the oil over medium heat, add the garlic, and stir-fry for a minute or two until the garlic starts to take color. Add the tomato purée, black pepper, and 3 tablespoons of the stock from the pan of beans. Mix well over a very low heat.

Drain the beans from the stock and add them to the pan of tomato mixture. Stir well to combine the ingredients and serve with the parsley scattered over the top.

## Refried beans

**ready in 30 minutes**

1 tablespoon olive oil

½ onion (approx. 2oz/60g) chopped

1 garlic clove, crushed

½ teaspoon cumin seeds

1 can (approx. 8oz/250g) pink, red, or cannelini beans, drained and rinsed

1 can (approx. 7½oz/225g) chopped tomatoes

¼ teaspoon chili powder

Freshly ground black pepper, to taste

Heat the oil in a heavy-bottomed saucepan and add the onion, garlic, and cumin seeds. Cook gently until the onions are soft and beginning to color. Add the beans, tomatoes, chili powder, and black pepper. Cook gently for 10–15 minutes, stirring and gently mashing down the beans with a fork. When the mixture is thick and beginning to come away from the sides of the pan, remove from the heat.

About 10 minutes before you are ready to serve the beans, heat a drizzle of olive oil in a small non-stick frying pan. Add the bean mix and flatten down into a cake. Cook for 5 minutes over medium-high heat to brown the base. Drizzle the top with a little more olive oil and slip the pan under a broiler for another 2–3 minutes to cook the top. Slide the bean cake on to a flat plate, cut in half and serve.

# Spiced rice

ready in **30** minutes

½ cup (100g) brown basmati rice

1 tablespoon olive oil

2 whole cardamom pods

⅓in (1cm) cinnamon stick

2 whole cloves

½ onion (approx. 1½oz/45g), finely chopped

1 cup (250ml) vegetable stock (*see p.149*)

Rinse the rice in a colander, put it in a bowl of fresh water, and let it stand until you are ready to use it.

Heat the oil in a heavy-bottomed saucepan over medium heat and add the spices whole. Stir them once or twice in the oil, then add the onions. Stir-fry until the onion begins to brown.

Drain the rice thoroughly and add it to the pan. Stir the mixture to coat the rice with oil before adding the hot stock. Bring to a boil, cover the pan, reduce the heat, and simmer for 25 minutes or until the rice is cooked. If all the stock has not been absorbed, turn up the heat and boil away the remainder before serving.

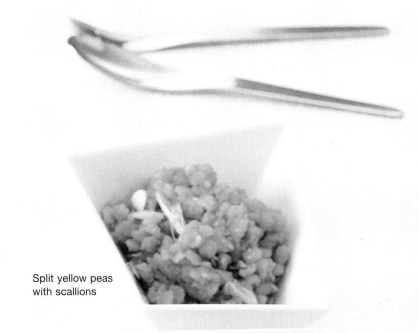

Split yellow peas with scallions

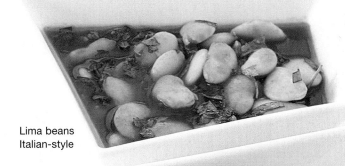

Lima beans Italian-style

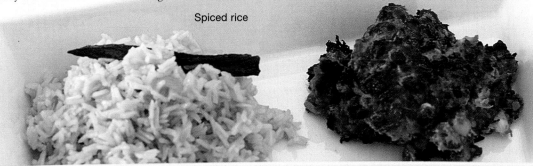

Refried beans

Spiced rice

# Menu ideas

# Handy meals

Be prepared. With just a few cans and dried goods you have good staples for a variety of filling, healthy dishes that will keep you from making poor food choices when you haven't been able to shop, or haven't the time to make a meal "from scratch."

## Fish, veggie & rice salad

*Make this dish with these ingredients:*

- **fish**　half a can of tuna, mackerel, or salmon, plus a few chopped anchovies

and

- **egg**　one hard-boiled egg

and

- **vegetables**　a tablespoon of frozen sweetcorn and a pinch of cumin

and

- **brown rice or quinoa**　a portion of brown rice for lunch, or quinoa for dinner (if using quinoa, increase the amount of vegetables)

## Tuna and mixed bean salad

*Make this salad with these ingredients:*

- **fish**　half a can of tuna, mackerel, or salmon

and

- **beans**　half a can of mixed beans, such as kidney or lima beans

and

- **vegetables**　a handfull of frozen peas, sweetcorn, or fava beans

and (if lunch-time)

- **quinoa**　one portion of quinoa, couscous, or bulgar wheat

## Vegetable soup

*Make this soup into a balanced meal with these ingredients:*

- **soup**　one can of vegetable-based soup, such as tomato or pumpkin

and

- **beans**　half a can of chickpeas, lentils, cannellini, or black-eye beans

and (if lunch-time)

- **bread**　one thick slice of whole-wheat or rye bread

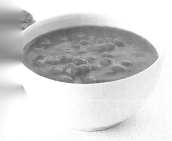

Vegetable soup

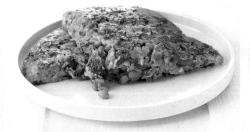

Omelet

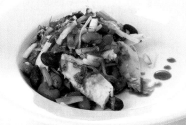

Tuna and mixed bean salad

## Vegetable chili

*Make this filling chili with these ingredients:*

- **quick tomato sauce**   half a portion of tomato sauce (*see p.143*) or ratatouille (*see p.96*)

  and

- **beans**   half a can of red kidney or black-eye beans

  and

- **flavors and spices**   one onion, chopped, and some chili powder

  and (if lunchtime)

- **brown rice**   a portion of brown rice

## Quick ragout

*Make this tomato dish with these ingredients:*

- **ratatouille**   half a can of ratatouille, or half a portion (*see p.96*)

  and

- **flavors and spices**   one chopped onion and some dried herbs

  and

- **goat cheese or shrimp**   a palm-sized piece of goat cheese, or a handful of frozen shrimp

  and (if lunchtime)

- **pasta**   a portion of corn, buckwheat, or whole-wheat pasta

## Omelet

*Make this quick omelet with these ingredients:*

- **eggs**   two eggs

  and

- **vegetables**   a teaspoon of pesto mixed with half a can of chopped plum tomatoes or half a jar of roasted sweet peppers, chopped

  or

- **beans**   half a can of flageleot, cannellini, or black-eye beans

# Pasta and pesto

This dish's carbohydrate:protein balance means that it is best served at lunchtime. If you prefer, make it with 4oz (125g) of quinoa cooked in stock, in place of the pasta. Serves two.

ready in **20** minutes

125g (4oz) buckwheat noodles, or whole-wheat pasta

2 eggs

1 tablespoon chopped fresh herbs (such as basil, parsley, and oregano)

3 tablespoons pesto (*see p.69*)

10 sun-dried tomatoes in oil, drained and sliced into ribbons

Freshly ground black pepper, to taste

Cook the pasta according to the instructions on the package. Drain into a colander and tip back into the empty pan to keep warm.

While the pasta is cooking, make a flat omelet with the eggs, flavored with mixed herbs (*see egg ribbons with cumin rice, p.139*). When the omelet is cooked, slide it from the pan on to a plate. When it is cool, roll up and cut into ribbons about ¼in (½cm) wide.

Stir the pesto into the pasta, add the tomatoes and black pepper, and serve with the egg ribbons on top.

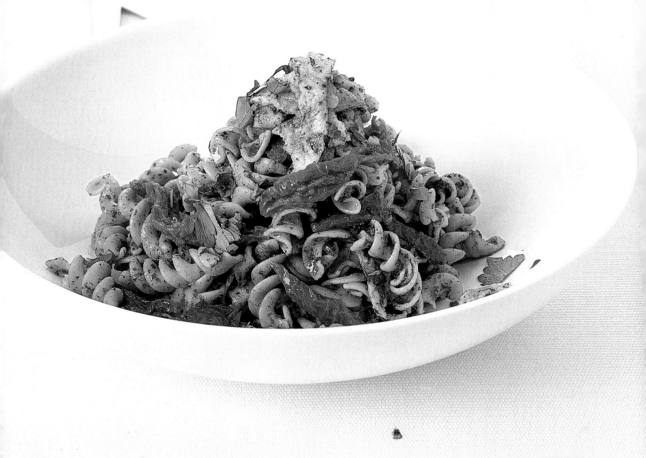

# Chickpea and ratatouille stew

**LUNCH OR DINNER**

This stew makes a filling meal on its own, and is delicious served either hot or cold. Put any leftovers in a blender if you want to make a smooth, healthy dip. Serves two.

**ready in 10 minutes**

1 tablespoon olive oil

1 small onion, sliced

13oz (400g) ratatouille (*see p.96*)

1 can (approx. 13oz/400g) chickpeas, drained and rinsed

Juice of 1 lemon

1 teaspoon paprika

Heat the oil in a heavy-bottomed saucepan over medium-low heat, add the onion, and cook gently until it begins to soften and turn opaque. Add the ratatouille, mix well, and heat through for a few minutes. Add the chickpeas, lemon juice, and paprika. Simmer everything together for a few more minutes to warm it through, then serve.

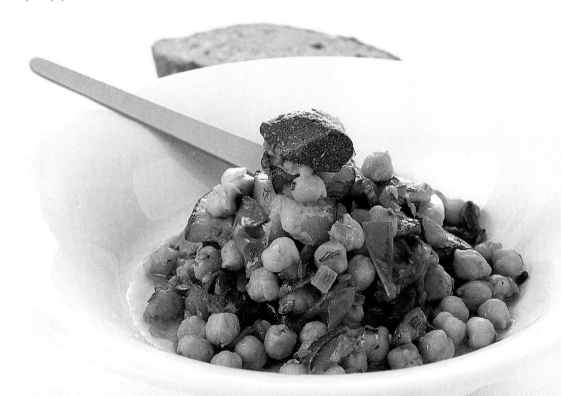

### SERVING IDEAS

**For lunch** Serve with a slice of whole-wheat bread, or some brown rice.

**For dinner** Stir in some frozen spinach to boost the complex carbohydrate ratio.

# Tuna and mixed bean salad

**LUNCH OR DINNER**

This salad can be made very quickly using ingredients from the pantry with fresh herbs and cucumber, if you have any. Serves two.

**ready in 10 minutes**

2 tablespoons olive oil

1 tablespoon lemon juice

1 tablespoon water

1 teaspoon tomato purée

1 teaspoon soy sauce

1 teaspoon Thai fish sauce, if available

1 can (10oz/300g) mixed beans, drained and rinsed

1 can (6oz/175g) solid-pack tuna in spring water, drained and broken into chunks

½ small red onion, finely sliced

½ small cucumber, diced (optional)

Fresh green herbs, such as parsley, cilantro, or marjoram, to garnish (optional)

Put the olive oil, lemon juice, water, tomato purée, soy sauce, and fish sauce in a salad bowl and mix together with a fork. Mix in the beans, then fold in the tuna chunks carefully so that they do not break up. Top with the raw onion.

Cucumbers add a refreshing coolness to this salad, if you have any, add small cubes of it to the salad before the tuna. Garnish with freshly chopped herbs if they are available.

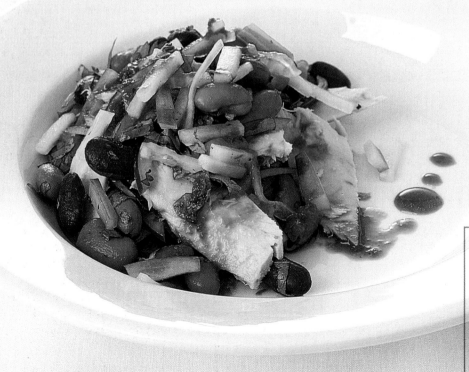

**SERVING IDEAS**

**For lunch** Add a spoonful of brown rice.

**For dinner** If you have any other salad vegetables, such as tomatoes, celery, or sweet peppers, chop them up and add them before the tuna.

# Egg ribbons with cumin rice

This lunch is simple to prepare and extremely versatile. If you don't have eggs available, try chicken strips or canned fish. Serves two.

**ready in 30 minutes**

**SERVING IDEA**

**For lunch** If you have any salad greens in the refrigerator serve them on the side drizzled with balsamic vinegar.

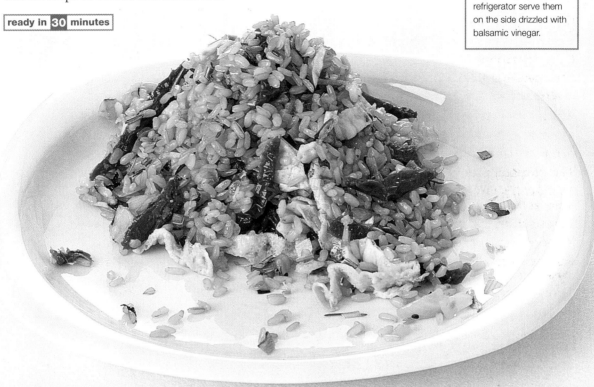

1 teaspoon olive oil

1 small onion (approx. 3½oz/100g), chopped

1 teaspoon cumin seeds

5oz (150g) brown rice

1½ cups (12fl oz/350ml) hot vegetable stock (*see p.149*)

2 eggs

Mixed herbs or spices (whatever you have in the kitchen)

Freshly ground black pepper, to taste

8 sun-dried tomatoes in oil, cut into strips

Chopped fresh parsley (optional)

Heat the olive oil in a saucepan over medium-low heat, add the onion and cook gently until soft but not colored. Add the cumin and stir for 1 minute. Add the rice, stir to coat with the oil, pour in the hot stock and cover. Bring to a boil, reduce the heat, and simmer for 30 minutes, until the stock is absorbed and the rice is tender.

Beat the eggs in a bowl, and add a good pinch of any dried herbs or spices you may have and some black pepper. Wipe the inside of a small nonstick skillet with a little oil, heat the pan over medium-high heat, and pour in the egg mixture. Cook the egg mixture quickly, without stirring it, to make a flat omelet. When the omelet is cool, roll it up and cut into strips about ¼in (½cm) wide.

Stir the tomatoes and egg ribbons into the rice and serve garnished with parsley, if you have any.

# Omelet with beans

This splendidly filling omelet is based on common pantry ingredients and is quick to make, so you can sit down to a satisfying meal within minutes of getting home from work. Serves two.

ready in **10** minutes

### SERVING IDEAS

**For lunch** Keep the preparation time to a minimum by serving with a hefty slice of whole-wheat or rye bread.

**For dinner** Serve with a few steamed snow peas, or a selection of green vegetables.

4 eggs

2 heaping teaspoons Dijon mustard

1 teaspoon dried mixed herbs

Freshly ground black pepper, to taste

1 can (approx. 7oz/200g) chopped tomatoes

Cooking spray

½ can (approx. 7oz/200g) flageolet or cannellini beans, drained and rinsed

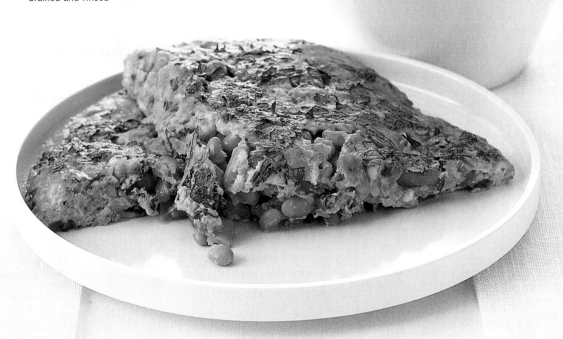

Break the eggs into a bowl and whisk them with the mustard, dried herbs, and black pepper. Mix in the chopped tomatoes.

Spray a nonstick skillet with cooking spray and heat over medium heat. Pour in the egg mixture, spreading it evenly over the bottom of the pan. Scatter the beans over the top and cook until the bottom is set and turning golden. Put the pan under the broiler for 3–4 minutes until the top is just set and golden in color, then serve.

# Lentils with onion and tomatoes

LUNCH OR **DINNER**

Cut down on the preparation time by using canned lentils, if available, as in the Lemon spinach soup (*see p.88*). Lentils are a great source of protein, fiber, and vitamins. Serves two.

ready in **30** minutes

½ cup (125g) French lentils

1½ cups (350ml) vegetable stock (*see p.149*)

1 tablespoon olive oil

1 onion, finely sliced

1 garlic clove, chopped

1 can (7½oz/225g) chopped tomatoes

1 heaping teaspoon tomato purée

1 teaspoon dried mixed herbs

Juice of ½ lemon

Place the lentils in a heavy-bottomed saucepan and pour in enough vegetable stock to cover them well. Bring to a boil, cover the pan, reduce the heat, and simmer for about 25 minutes, or until the lentils are cooked. Check the liquid level from time to time and add more hot stock, if necessary. Drain the cooked lentils.

While the lentils are cooking, heat the oil in a heavy-bottomed pan over medium heat, add the onion and garlic, and cook until softened and golden. Add the tomatoes and their juice, along with the tomato purée and dried herbs to the pan, mix well, and bring to the simmering point. Stir the lentils and lemon juice into the onion and tomato mixture and serve.

---

### SERVING IDEAS

**For lunch** Serve with a spoonful of brown rice or some whole-wheat bread.

**For dinner** Stir in some frozen spinach.

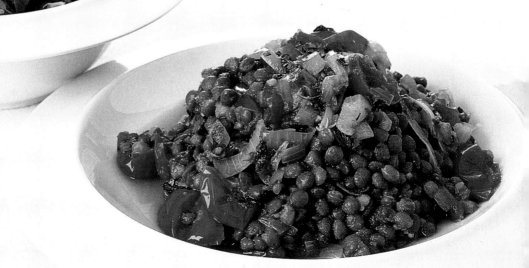

# With just a can of tomatoes ...

Here are four great recipes, all with a can of tomatoes as their main ingredient. They are the perfect answer to the dilemma of a nearly-empty pantry. The quick tomato sauce is excellent with grilled chicken or fish and will keep for several days in an airtight container in the fridge. Each recipe serves two.

## Baked eggs on tomatoes and peppers

ready in **25** minutes

3 tablespoons olive oil

1 onion (approx. 7oz/200g), coarsely chopped

1 garlic clove, crushed and chopped

1 red pepper, cored, seeded and chopped

1 yellow pepper, cored, seeded and chopped

1 can (14oz/400g) chopped tomatoes

2–3 tablespoons chopped fresh parsley

Freshly ground black pepper, to taste

2 eggs

Preheat the oven to 350°F/180°C/gas mark 4. Heat the oil in a heavy-bottomed saucepan over medium heat. Add the onion and garlic and cook for about 3 minutes until transparent. Add the peppers and cook for an additional 5 minutes, until they begin to soften. Add the tomatoes, parsley and pepper and simmer everything together for an additional 5 minutes, stirring often.

When the vegetable mixture is cooked, pour it into an ovenproof dish, break the eggs on top, and bake in the preheated oven for about 10 minutes, or until the egg whites are just set. Serve immediately.

## Quick tomato soup

ready in **10** minutes

1 recipe quantity quick tomato sauce (*see opposite*)

1 cup (250ml) chicken or vegetable stock (*see p.149*)

1 tablespoon plain yogurt

Fresh basil, to garnish

Put the quick tomato sauce and stock in a blender and blend to make a soup.

Pour into a saucepan and heat to the simmering point. Divide between two bowls and put a swirl of yogurt on top of each. Serve garnished with the basil.

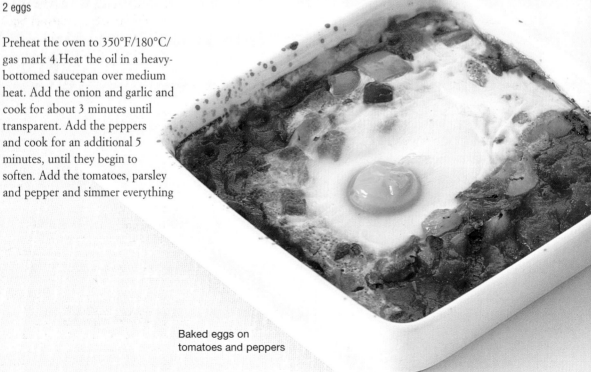

Baked eggs on
tomatoes and peppers

## Tomato and lime juice drink

ready in **5** minutes

1 can (13oz/400g) tomatoes

Juice of 1 lime

Dash of Worcestershire sauce

Put all the ingredients in a blender and blend thoroughly to make a zesty and refreshing tomato drink.

Note: An ounce of vodka turns this tomato drink into a cocktail very like the famous Bloody Mary.

## Quick tomato sauce

ready in **20** minutes

2 tablespoons olive oil

1 onion (approx. 5oz/150g), finely chopped

1 garlic clove, finely chopped

1 can (7oz/200g) chopped tomatoes

1 tablespoon lemon juice

1 tablespoon tomato purée

Freshly ground black pepper, to taste

2 tablespoons chopped fresh herbs, such as parsley, cilantro, or basil

Heat the oil in a heavy-bottomed saucepan over medium-low heat and add the onion and garlic. Cook gently for about 5 minutes, until softened but not colored. Add the tomatoes, lemon juice, tomato purée, and black pepper. Bring to a boil and simmer for 10–15 minutes, until the sauce has thickened. Stir in the chopped fresh herbs.

Tomato and lime juice drink

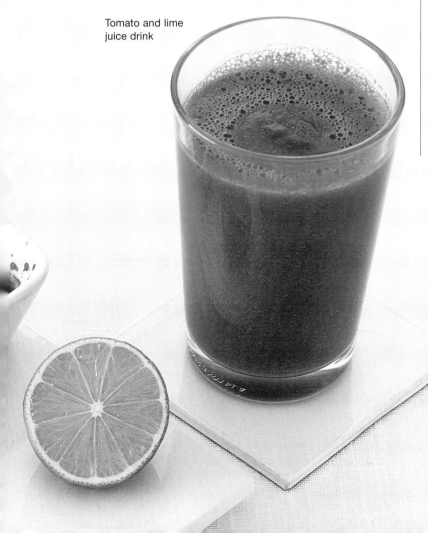

### SERVING IDEAS

**For lunch** The soup makes a great lunch, hot or cold, accompanied by whole-wheat bread or crackers. Add some pulses, tofu, or chicken to provide the protein.

**For dinner** The baked eggs recipe is a meal in itself, or you could liven up a chicken or fish fillet and steamed vegetables with a spoonful or two of the quick tomato sauce.

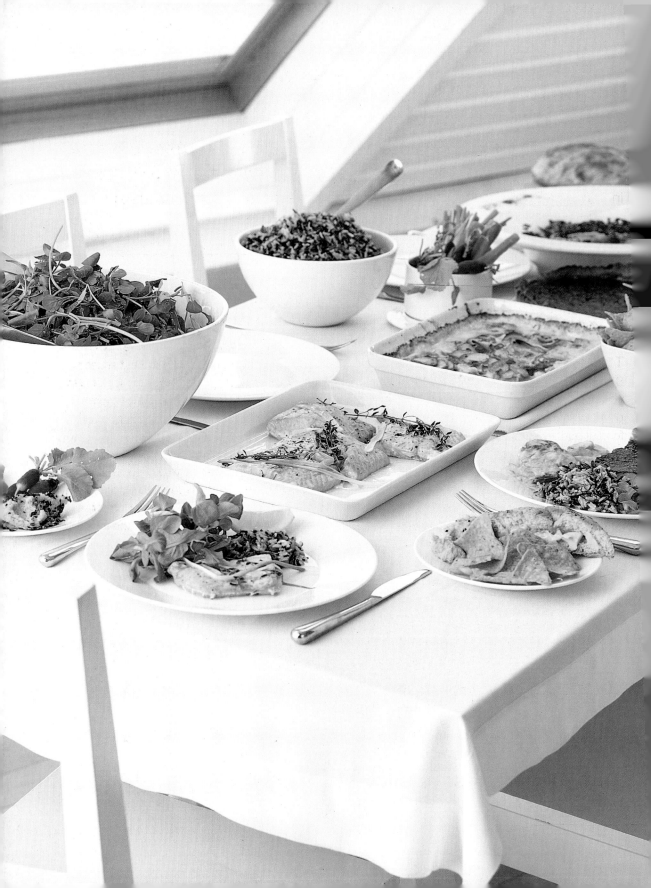

# Eating out

If you have a mantra for eating out—whether at a restaurant, a friend's house, a work function, or even on vacation—it should be "Where's the protein?" Keep that in mind, and remember the 10 principles, and you can navigate any situation.

There are many strategies to ensure that, whatever the occasion, you won't need to sabotage your weight control to enjoy it. Simple tactics such as drinking a few glasses of water and having a little snack before you go out will ensure that you avoid hunger and blood-glucose lows.

## Think strong
Sometimes a slight shift in mindset is involved. If you've been brought up to eat everything on your plate, for instance, you must adjust to leaving food. If portion sizes are enormous, you can gauge how much to eat using your hands.

Don't feel intimidated about making requests in restaurants either: If you want extra green vegetables instead of the mashed potatoes your dish is served with, just ask. Sauces and dressings can be served separately, keeping you in control of how much you eat. The current allergy-aware climate is becoming more and more receptive to individual requirements.

You might want to indulge in "stealth-dieting." Don't actually tell anyone you're watching what you eat, and then you'll be spared the I-know-better advice, the conspiratorial attempts to lead you astray, and the evenings spent discussing every diet someone's mother, neighbor, or sister has done and how well it worked for them.

## Where there's a will ...
Desserts are a problem, so you will need a little willpower here, or apply the 80:20 rule (see pp.12–13). And don't be tempted to skip a meal earlier in the day to "save" the calories for your evening out—this will only end up upsetting your blood-glucose levels (see pp.16–17).

### DRINKING AND DIETING

Alcohol is a simple carbohydrate that is easily absorbed into the blood, raising levels of blood-glucose quite quickly and probably sending you over the insulin threshold. Therefore, I suggest you drink alcohol only with your meal, not before, since the presence of food will slow down the glucose conversion to some extent. I know from my own experience that a couple of drinks before dinner may be part of the evening, but your chances of making good food choices afterward are decreased as you feel more relaxed. This doesn't mean you have to abstain—just be aware.

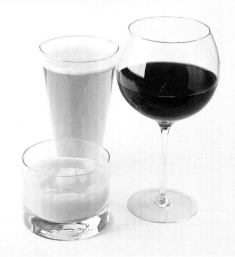

# Hosting a dinner party

If you're hosting the dinner, you're in control, which is perfect. I believe that it is entirely possible to feed your guests from the Food Doctor Daily Diet without any of them realizing they're on your "diet" with you.

For example, start with a soup, or crudités with dips (perhaps set these out for people to graze on beforehand—then you won't feel obliged to offer chips). Your main course could be almost any recipe from this book, such as the Seared tuna with cinnamon (*see p.128*), or the Chicken with summer herbs (*see p.123*). Serve with vegetables, salads, or spreads and guests won't even notice the absence of starchy carbohydrates. If you want, of course, you can serve these as well, and simply abstain yourself unless it's lunchtime. Dessert is harder, since you don't want to be eating sugary food: Perhaps a very dark chocolate mousse that has little added sugar, or a fresh fruit salad with yogurt rather than cream. Or serve cheese—just avoid the crackers yourself.

If you present dishes in separate serving bowls, your guests can help themselves to what they want, and you can stick to the Food Doctor plan easily and without fuss.

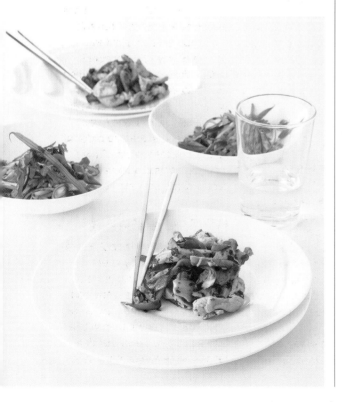

# Dining out at a friend's

This can be slightly tricky, since you are not in control of the cooking. You are also unable to control what time you will eat, so I suggest having a small snack before you leave the house, even if it's just a rice cake with a protein spread, or some vegetables and hummus or fish dip.

You can't dictate what you are served either, but you can control what you actually eat. Usually somewhere within whatever is served there will be a protein and some vegetables together with the necessary complex carbohydrates. You have the tools to assess and create a suitable meal from what you are served: The food group ratios, the portion sizes according to your hand size, and the mantra "Where's the protein?" Leave what doesn't make the cut on the side of your plate—whoever is providing the food won't be offended. If they ask why you didn't eat whatever it is you have left, just say that you are full and have eaten enough.

If, unfortunately, you have been offered a main course based on simple carbohydrates (such as a risotto), or you feel that you want to eat more than usual or eat in a way that wouldn't fit in with my plan, then be honest with yourself about it and do not feel guilty. See this as a "20 percent moment" (*see pp.12–13*). You have made good food choices 80 percent of the time, so you can relax the rules for 20 percent. Assuming you don't do it every day, you won't suddenly regain the weight you have lost.

# Restaurants

The great thing about eating in restaurants is that you can order what you want from the menu, as long as you bear the 10 principles in mind. If you think about what type of food is offered, then I am sure you can apply the principles almost anywhere (*see box, opposite*).

Whether you eat out because your job demands it, your partner loves it, or because you choose to, it's really easy to follow the Food Doctor plan. I have to eat out a fair amount, and find it simple to follow my own principles. I don't have any special willpower or self-control—just the confidence to eat in a way that makes sense.

When sizing up the menu, remember the mantra "Where's the protein?". If there isn't any, then the dish is unlikely to fit the bill. Don't be afraid to be specific about what you want to eat—remember, you're the customer. And, of course, always avoid the bread basket!

# Drinking parties

This is tricky for healthy eating, not just due to the alcohol intake, the empty stomach, and the likelihood of poor food choices following later in the evening. An average evening of drinks, possibly with snacks, followed by a late meal, plays havoc with your blood-glucose levels, and insulin production is pretty much inevitable.

Minimize the dangers by drinking plenty of water before you go out, and eating a small snack (*see pp.62–63*) to steady your blood-glucose levels. Try to avoid snacks such as chips and salted nuts, sticking to olives or raw, unsalted nuts if you can. Stick to white or red wine rather than liquor or beer, which have higher GI scores.

# Vacations

Traditional dieters all too often lose weight before a vacation so they will feel comfortable in their bikinis or bathing suits. Sadly, once the vacation feeling kicks in, we all know that we will probably abandon our good intentions and eat and eat and eat (I bet there will be someone who says "Go on, you're on vacation, you deserve it—after all, look how good you have been.")

Remind yourself that it's the vacation you deserve, not weight gain, so follow the 10 principles and you will be fine. By all means have fun and try new foods, but you will be back on the diet treadmill if you just overeat and then have to diet again once you are home.

## DIFFERENT RESTAURANTS, DIFFERENT CUISINES, SAME TACTICS

In almost any type of restaurant, there will be something on the menu to fit the 10 principles. Remember portion control, too.

### FRENCH RESTAURANTS

French food is easy—onion soup and a grilled piece of fish or meat, with some potatoes and vegetables is typical, and certainly what I would order. The trick is to feel free to ask for just a couple of new potatoes, rather than let the restaurant choose the portion size for you.

### ITALIAN RESTAURANTS

You don't have to have pasta or a pizza, since even the most basic pizza chain will have salads. You could start with a mozzarella and tomato salad, followed by seafood pasta. Or grilled veal with vegetables. The protein doesn't have to be in both the starter and the main course—just consider how much protein you are eating in the whole meal. This means that if you want some bread at the start of the meal, then this counts as part of your carbohydrate intake. If you choose pasta, then ask for extra seafood and less pasta—restaurants are there to serve food, so never be afraid to ask for what you want.

### INDIAN RESTAURANTS

Indian food is overly dependent on carbohydrates, so you must be especially aware at an Indian restaurant. The typical meal starts with papadums, which are made from lentil flour. This contains protein, but only a little, so papadums hardly count towards your protein quota. A typical order might previously have been a chicken dish with a sauce, some naan bread, and some rice. If you follow the Food Doctor plan and apply the 10 principles, then you can still start with the papadums, but follow it instead with tandoori chicken or fish, accompanied by vegetables, and a lentil or chickpea dish.

### ASIAN RESTAURANTS

Asian food is often heavy on rice and noodles, but that doesn't mean you have to avoid this cuisine altogether. You could order chicken satay to start, then have a duck or tofu curry and some rice. However, ask for extra chicken (make a scene if you have to), and share one order of rice with someone else. This way you can still achieve 40% protein while enjoying the meal.

### MEXICAN RESTAURANTS

This cuisine is very carbohydrate-oriented so ensure you eat something before you arrive at the restaurant. Have a few corn chips, then try some chicken or beef tacos or enchiladas with a side salad to achieve the ideal ratio of protein to carbohydrates.

# Useful recipes and ingredients

## Five-spice paste

This paste is a little easier to use than the powder (*see below*) because it can be blended easily. If neither the powder or the paste is available, you could substitute a small pinch of cinnamon and clove to the dish you are cooking, although it will taste quite the same.

2 teaspoons five-spice powder

1 tablespoon soy sauce

2 garlic cloves, crushed

Blend all the ingredients to a paste. It can be stored for up to a week in a screw-topped jar in the fridge.

## Five-spice powder

This seasoning originated in China and takes its name from the five flavors included in it (salty, sour, bitter, pungent, and sweet). Sometimes it can be extended to seven with the addition of dried ginger, cardamom, or licorice. Both the powder and paste (*see above*) are quite pungent so use sparingly.

6 star anise

1 tablespoon Szechuan pepper

1 tablespoon ground fennel seeds

2 teaspoons cloves

2 teaspoons ground cassia or cinnamon

Grind all the ingredients in a blender until very fine. Sieve and store in an airtight container.

## Green tapenade

Tapenade is a spread or accompaniment from southern France. This recipe is based on green olives, but black olives can be used if that's what you have available.

1 cup (150g) green olives, pitted and finely chopped

6–7 anchovy fillets, rinsed and dried

1 small tablespoon capers

Olive oil

Lemon juice

Put the olives, anchovies, and capers in a bowl or and mash them well together. Add a dash of olive oil and a few drops of lemon juice to taste. Store in the fridge in a screw-top jar.

## Herbes de Provence

The herbs in the mixture vary considerably but usually include four or five of the following: Sage, parsley, rosemary, hyssop, thyme, marjoram, fennel seed, savory, and bay—plus basil and lavender. Vary the amounts and herb choices to suit your own taste.

3 tablespoons dried thyme

2 tablespoons dried marjoram

1 teaspoon dried rosemary

1 tablespoon dried savory

1 teaspoon dried lavender flowers

Crumble or grind the herbs and store in an air-tight container for 2–3 months.

## Horseradish sauce

A popular, quickly prepared substitute for store-bought horseradish sauce is a mixture of finely grated fresh horseradish and sour cream, or cream and a little lemon juice or vinegar. This sauce is commonly used for fish, poultry, or vegetables such as zucchinis and beets. Makes enough for four servings.

½ cup (125g) plain yogurt

2 tablespoons horseradish, freshly grated

2 tablespoons chopped fresh dill

Freshly ground black pepper, to taste

Mix all the ingredients together in a bowl. Store covered in the refrigerator until needed.

If you wish to serve it warm, heat it over a double boiler but make sure it doesn't because this will make it curdle.

## Soy sauce

Soy sauce is extracted from boiled soy beans that have been fermented with barley or wheat, then salted and fermented again. Choose a light sauce if possible for use in cooking, ideally in combination with other liquids such as wine or stock, and a dark sauce for a condiment to be sprinkled sparingly (it is very salty) over finished dishes.

# Fish stock

To make a good fish stock, ask the grocer for trimmings—the heads without gills, fins, or bones—of white fish such as monkfish, cod, whiting, and (because their bones are full of gelatine) turbot and sole. Avoid oily fish like mackerel and herring. Makes approximately 7 cups (2 liters).

2–3lb (1–1½kg) white fish trimmings

1 onion, peeled and sliced

1 carrot, sliced

1 small leek (white part only), sliced

1 stick celery, chopped

1 sprig of dill

1 sprig of parsley

1 bay leaf

10–12 black peppercorns

1½ cups (350ml) dry white wine

6 cups (1.4 liters) water

Put all the ingredients in a large saucepan and bring slowly to a boil, skimming the surface until the liquid is clear. As soon as the stock has reached the boiling point, turn down the heat, partially cover the pan, and let simmer for 30 minutes. Do not let the stock reach a full boil or let it simmer for more than 30 minutes, or it will become sticky.

Immediately strain the stock through a muslin-lined colander or sieve. The stock may be used at once or cooled and stored in the refrigerator for one day only before using it. Try freezing stock in an ice-cube tray so that you have convenient portions that you can add to smaller dishes.

# Vegetable stock

Most root vegetables, onions, leeks, and celery are good basic ingredients for a vegetable stock. Avoid strong green vegetables such as cabbage, broccoli, spinach, or Brussels sprouts, since they give stock too strong a flavor and color. The whole garlic bulb in this stock may sound like a lot, but it adds a deliciously subtle flavor. Makes approximately 5 cups (1.5 liters). It can be frozen in handy portion sizes when it has cooled.

2 potatoes or 1 parsnip, roughly chopped

2 carrots, roughly chopped

1 large onion, quartered

1 stick celery, roughly chopped

1 garlic bulb, unpeeled (optional)

1 bay leaf

1 large sprig fresh thyme or ½ teaspoon dried thyme

Large sprig parsley

6–8 black peppercorns

7 cups (1.6 liters) water

Put all the ingredients into a large saucepan. Bring slowly to a boil, then reduce the heat, partially cover and simmer gently for about 2 hours.

While the stock is simmering, line a colander or large sieve with a piece of muslin and set it over a large bowl. When the stock has finished cooking, pour it through the muslin-lined colander into the bowl. Discard the contents of the colander. Cover the bowl and set aside to cool thoroughly before storing in the refrigerator. It will keep for 3–4 days in the refrigerator, or you can freeze it.

# Tamarind paste

Tamarind pods look like long dates and the pulp inside, which has a distinctive sour, fruity flavor, is used as a souring agent in Indian and Southeast Asian cookery. Tamarind is usually found in the form of a paste. If it is not available, use lemon juice or wine vinegar instead.

# Thai fish sauce

Often labeled simply "fish sauce," this is sold in the Oriental foods section of most supermarkets. Thai fish sauce is a very salty, thin, brown liquid used in Malay and Thai cooking, where it is called "nam pla."

It is made by fermenting fish or shrimps with salt and soy. The liquid that is drained off from the fermentation is the fish sauce. If it is not available, anchovy essence makes an acceptable substitute.

# Tofu

This ingredient of Chinese and Japanese cooking is made from puréed soy beans. Bean curd is soft and white, with a cheeselike texture that ranges from firm to silken. It is high in protein and very low in fat.

Firm tofu is used largely as a salad ingredient, added in bite-sized cubes. Silken tofu is the best tofu for cooking with. It is used largely for blending into other ingredients to make sauces.

Tofu is also available marinated or smoked. These are best used in salads or stir-fries.

# Smart food choices

These charts give you a simple overview to help you make the best possible food choices. They are based on a range of criteria, including antioxidant properties, levels of essential fatty acids, fiber content, and rating on the Glycemic Index (GI).

The GI rating is, in effect, a measure of the sugar content of carbohydrates and a guide to how quickly the body converts that sugar to glucose. The quicker the conversion, the higher the GI score. Carbohydrates fall into two categories: simple and complex. Simple carbohydrates have had their fiber removed, while the fiber of complex carbohydrates remains intact. Fiber helps slow down the process of converting food into glucose, so foods high in fiber have lower GI scores. Foods high in sugars and low in fiber convert rapidly into blood-glucose and therefore have relatively high GI scores.

## Protein profiles

| | MEAT & POULTRY | |
|---|---|---|
| **Ideal choice**<br>These foods are all complete proteins and are therefore the best choice. | Calf's liver<br>Chicken, skinless<br>Lamb's liver<br>Turkey, skinless<br>Veal | |
| **Good choice**<br>You can include these food choices frequently as part of a healthy diet. | | |
| **Adequate choice**<br>Eat these foods occasionally. | Bacon<br>Beef<br>Duck, skinless<br>Game<br>Ham | Hamburger<br>Lamb<br>Pork |

## Carbohydrate profiles

| | GRAIN-BASED FOODS | FRUITS | |
|---|---|---|---|
| **Ideal choice**<br>The complex carbohydrates at this level are ideal choices because they supply high levels of energy for a sustained period. They are all broken down slowly into glucose by the body so they have a low GI score. | Barley flakes<br>Bran flakes<br>Buckwheat flour or flakes<br>Millet<br>Oatmeal or oat flakes<br>Rye bread (wholegrain) or rye flakes | Apples<br>Apricots (fresh)<br>Blackberries<br>Cranberries<br>Currants<br>Grapefruit<br>Lemons<br>Limes<br>Pears | Plums<br>Strawberries |
| **Good choice**<br>The foods in this category have a medium GI score and so they provide reasonably good levels of energy at a fairly steady rate. | Couscous<br>Granola bars containing nuts<br>Pasta, e.g. corn, buckwheat, or whole-wheat<br>Pumpernickel bread<br>Rice, brown<br>Whole-wheat bread | Blueberries<br>Cherries<br>Grapes, white or<br>red<br>Loganberries<br>Mandarins<br>Mangoes | Oranges<br>Papayas<br>Peaches<br>Pineapple<br>Tangerines |
| **Adequate choice**<br>These foods have a relatively high GI score and provide only short-term energy, so do not include them too frequently in your eating plan. | Bagels<br>Breadsticks<br>Breakfast cereals (unsweetened)<br>French bread<br>Soda bread<br>Sourdough bread | Bananas<br>Dried fruit<br>Figs<br>Prunes | |

| DAIRY | VEGETARIAN | FISH | | | |
|---|---|---|---|---|---|
| Duck eggs<br>Hen's eggs<br>Quail's eggs | Nuts (raw)<br>Quinoa<br>Pulses, e.g. cannellini<br>  beans, lima beans,<br>  chickpeas, lentils<br>Seeds, e.g. pumpkin,<br>  sesame, and sunflower<br>Tofu | Anchovies<br>Bluefish*<br>Bream<br>Brill<br>Carp*<br>Cod<br>Dover sole<br>Eel*<br>Grey Mullet* | Gurnard<br>Haddock<br>Hake<br>Halibut*<br>Herring*<br>Hoki<br>Lemon sole<br>Mackerel*<br>Mahi Mahi* | Marlin*<br>Monkfish<br>Orange roughy<br>Perch*<br>Plaice<br>Red mullet*<br>Salmon*<br>Sardine*<br>Sea bass | Sea bream<br>Skate<br>Sprat*<br>Swordfish*<br>Trout*<br>Tuna*<br>Turbot<br>Whitebait*<br>Whiting |
| Cottage cheese, low-fat<br>Goat cheese (hard or<br>  soft)<br>Yogurt, plain or low-fat | Baked beans<br>(unsweetened) | Lobster<br>Mussels<br>Scallops<br>Shrimp<br>Squid | | | |
| Butter, unsalted<br>Cheese, hard<br>Sour cream<br>Milk, whole or low-fat<br>Ricotta cheese<br>Yogurt, full-fat | | | | | |

*Also a good source of omega-3 fats

| COOKED VEGETABLES | | RAW FOODS | | DRINKS |
|---|---|---|---|---|
| Artichokes<br>Asparagus<br>Green beans<br>Bok choi<br>Broccoli<br>Brussels sprouts<br>Cabbage, red or<br>  green<br>Cauliflower | Kale<br>Leeks<br>Peppers, sweet red,<br>  orange or yellow<br>Onions<br>Spinach | Arugula<br>Bean sprouts<br>Celery<br>Chicory<br>Corn salad<br>Mushrooms<br>Peppers, sweet<br>red, orange, or<br>yellow | Spinach<br>Sprouted seeds<br>  and beans, e.g.<br>  alfalfa, mung<br>Tomatoes<br>Watercress | Vegetable juice |
| Carrots<br>Kidney beans<br>Pumpkin<br>Turnips<br>Yellow squash<br>Zucchini | | Avocados<br>Beets<br>Carrots<br>Celeriac<br>Olives<br>Peppers, sweet green<br>Radishes | | Fruit juice |
| Eggplant<br>Parsnips<br>Peas<br>Potatoes, baked,<br>  boiled, or mashed<br>Squash | Sweet potatoes<br>Yams | | | Beer<br>Liquor<br>Mixers<br>Wine |

# Glossary

### Adrenaline
A hormone secreted by the adrenal glands (located above the kidneys) in response to low blood-glucose levels, exercise, or stress. Adrenaline causes an increase in blood-glucose levels by breaking down stored glycogen to glucose in the liver, encouraging the release of fatty acids from body tissue, causing blood vessels to dilate, and increasing cardiac output.

### Amino acids
Amino acids form the basic constituents of proteins. There are nine essential amino acids that cannot be produced by the body and must be supplied by food, although the ninth is only considered essential for children.

### Blood-glucose levels
The concentration of glucose in the blood.

### Cardiovascular
Relating to the heart and blood vessels.

### Complex carbohydrate
A food containing insoluble fiber, which helps to slow down the process of digestion.

### Diuretic effect
Increases the rate of urination, generally decreasing water retention.

### Essential fats
Fats that are essential to the normal functioning of the body, but which cannot be created by the body and thus have to be derived from foods. Omega-3 essential fats are found in oily fish, such as salmon, mackerel, herring, tuna, and sardines, and also in flax and hemp seeds. Omega-6 oils are found in most seeds and nuts except peanuts.

### Famine mode
The point at which a dieter's metabolism senses a reduction in food intake and slows down to conserve energy in response to this "famine" situation.

### Fiber
Mostly derived from plant cell walls, fiber is not broken down by digestive enzymes but may be partly digested by beneficial bacteria in the intestines. Fiber is essential for good digestive health: Insoluble fiber provides bulk to the feces and thus helps to prevent constipation; soluble fiber helps to reduce blood-cholesterol levels and eliminate toxins and excess hormones.

### Free radical
A naturally occurring, short-lived, highly unstable molecule that is usually produced when chemical reactions occur in the body. In its search for stability, it will "steal" an electron from another molecule, causing it to become a free radical. This results in a cascade of free radical activity, which can result in the deterioration of tissue and degeneration associated with aging, cancer, Alzheimer's, Parkinson's disease, arthritis, and many other conditions. Stress, pollution, poor diet, excessive sun exposure, smoking, radiation, and illness all increase the buildup of free radicals.

### Glucose
A simple form of sugar, also known as a monosaccharide. It occurs naturally in various foods—for example, in some fruits—and is the body's main source of fuel. Carbohydrates are broken down into glucose by the body. However, body cells cannot use glucose without the help of insulin.

### Gluten
An insoluble protein group that is found in wheat, rye, barley, and oats. Gluten is the mixture of proteins, which includes gliadin, to which celiacs are intolerant.

### Glycemic index
The glycemic index (GI) ranks foods on a scale of 1–100 according to how they affect blood-glucose levels. It measures how much blood sugar increases in the two or three hours after eating. Foods that are broken down quickly during the process of digestion have the highest GI values (70 and above)—they make blood-glucose levels rise high quickly. Foods that are broken down slowly, releasing glucose gradually into the bloodstream, have low GI scores (under 55).

### Hydrochloric acid
Hydrochloric acid, or stomach acid, is the acid component of gastric juice. It plays a number of important roles in the process of digestion, including creating the right acidic environment for protein digestion to occur and killing many pathogens present in food.

### Insulin
The hormone insulin is produced by the pancreas and helps glucose to enter the body's cells where it is used up as fuel. Insulin is also a storage hormone in that it will cause any excess glucose that is not needed immediately for energy to be stored as glycogen in the liver or muscles, or converted to fat and stored in body tissue.

### Insulin threshold
The point at which the level of glucose in the body rises so high that it tips insulin production over optimum levels, thus encouraging glucose to be added to the body's fat stores.

### Insulin trigger
Factor that encourages glucose levels to rise, such as foods easily converted into glucose, but also caffeine, smoking, and stress.

### Irritable bowel syndrome (IBS)
Irritable bowel syndrome, also known as spastic colon, is a common disorder whereby the regular waves of muscular movement along the intestines become uncoordinated. This disruption, involving both the small intestine and

the colon, results in a variety of symptoms in all areas of the digestive tract, including intermittent diarrhea and constipation, cramplike abdominal pain, and swelling of the abdomen.

## Metabolic rate
The energy required to keep the body functioning while at rest.

## Metabolism
The "burning" of glucose in body cells to produce energy.

## Minerals
Substances, such as calcium, magnesium, and iron, that are naturally found in various foods and which are required by the body for the maintenance of good health. A balanced, healthy diet usually contains all the minerals the body requires.

## Nutrients
Vital substances required by all living organisms for survival.

## Organic produce
Food that has been produced using farming methods that severely restrict the use of artificial chemical fertilizers and pesticides, and animals reared without the routine use of drugs, antibiotics and wormers common in intensive livestock farming.

## Osteoporosis
A condition in which the density of bones declines, making them brittle and prone to fracture. The mineral calcium is essential for bone health.

## Protein
A complex compound, made of carbon, hydrogen, oxygen, nitrogen, and often sulphur, which is essential to all living things. Protein is required for growth and repair and is broken down into amino acids by the body.

## Saliva
An alkaline liquid secreted by the salivary glands into the mouth. Saliva lubricates food, which helps with the process of chewing and swallowing, and contains an enzyme that helps to break down the starch contained in foods. It also has antibacterial properties.

## Saturated fats
Saturated fats are primarily animal fats that are solid at room temperature. They are found in meat and dairy products. Coconut oil is the only vegetable oil that contains a significant amount of saturated fats. Saturated fats have been shown to raise the levels of "bad" LDL (low-density lipoprotein) cholesterol in the blood.

## Set point
The point at which the body's intake of food provides exactly the amount of glucose required for its day-to-day energy requirements.

## Simple carbohydrate
A food that yields simple sugars, which are broken down rapidly into glucose by the body.

## Stimulants
Substances, including caffeine, found in foods and drinks such as chocolate and soda that stimulate the production of adrenaline from the adrenal glands. Under normal circumstances, this release of adrenaline prepares the body for the "fight or flight" response, causing the heart to beat faster, among many other things (*see p.20*). If adrenaline is overproduced because stimulant foods have been consumed, this may lead to fatigue and blood-glucose imbalances in the body.

## Type 2 diabetes
*Diabetes mellitus* is a condition in which blood-glucose levels can become dangerously high because the body cannot utilize glucose properly. Excess blood-glucose levels (hyperglycemia) can result in long-term damage to the eyes, kidneys, nerves, heart, and major arteries. There are two principal types of diabetes: Insulin-dependent Type 1 diabetes, and non-insulin-dependent Type 2 diabetes, also known as adult-onset diabetes.

In Type 2 diabetes, either the body cannot make enough insulin, or cell receptors do not respond to insulin (also known as insulin resistance). This type of diabetes usually occurs in people over the age of 40, although it is becoming increasingly common in the younger population due to an increase in high-sugar, refined-carbohydrate diets—even teenagers are now being diagnosed.

## Vitamins
Groups of complex organic substances, found in many different foods, that are essential in small amounts for the normal functioning of the body. There are 13 vitamins and, with the exception of vitamin D and niacin which can be generated by the body, vitamins must be obtained from your diet. A varied diet will contain adequate amounts of all the vitamins.

## Yeast
A single-celled organism used in some food industry processes such as baking, brewing, and winemaking. Some yeasts become pathogens once inside the body (*Candida albicans*, for example) and may cause infection in any open canal in the body, such as the vagina, ear, or mouth. Excess sugar, alcohol, stress, or antibiotics can cause a proliferation in pathogenic yeasts.

# Useful addresses and websites

*Please note that, because of the fast-changing nature of the internet, some websites may be out of date by the time you read this.*

## ORGANIZATIONS IN THE US

**The American College of Cardiology**
Heart House
9111 Old Georgetown Road
Bethesda, MD 20814-1699
tel: (800) 253-4636
www.acc.org

**American College of Gastroenterology**
P.O. Box 3099
Alexandria, VA 22302
tel: (703) 820-7400
www.acg.gi.org

**American Diabetes Association**
1701 North Beauregard Street
Alexandria, VA 23311
tel: (800) DIABETES
www.diabetes.org

**American Dietetic Association**
120 South Riverside Plaza
Suite 2000
Chicago, IL 60606-6995
tel: (800) 877-1600
www.eatright.org

**American Gastroenterological Association**
4930 Del Ray Avenue
Bethesda, MD 20814
tel: (301) 654-2055
www.gastro.org

**American Heart Association National Center**
7272 Greenville Avenue
Dallas, TX 75321
tel: (800) AHA-USA-1
www.americanheart.org

**Asthma and Allergy Foundation of America**
1233 20th Street NW
Suite 402
Washington, DC 20036
tel: (800) 7-ASTHMA
www.aafa.org

**Celiac Disease Foundation**
13521 Ventura Boulevard #1
Studio City, CA 91604
tel: (818) 990-2354
www.celiac.org

**Celiac Spruce Association**
P.O. Box 31700
Omaha, NE 68131-0700
tel: (402) 558-0600
www.csaceliacs.org

**Crohn's and Colitis Foundation of America**
386 Park Avenue South, 17th Floor
New York, NY 10016
tel: (800) 932-2423
www.ccfa.org

**Food and Nutrition Information Center**
National Agricultural Library, Room 105
10301 Baltimore Avenue
Beltsville, MD 20705-2351
tel: (301)-504-5719
www.nal.usda.gov/fnic

**Irritable Bowel Syndrome Association**
1440 Whalley Avenue #145
New Haven, CT 06515
www.ibsassociation.org

**National Digestive Diseases Information Clearinghouse**
2 Information Way
Bethesda, MD 20892-3570
tel: (800)) 891-5389
www.digestive.niddk.nih.gov

**National Heart, Lung, and Blood Institute**
P.O. Box 30105
Bethesda, MD 20824-0105
tel: (301) 592-8573
www.nhlbi.nih.gov

**National Osteoporosis Foundation**
1232 22nd Street NW
Washington, DC 20037-1292
tel: (202) 223-2226
www.nof.org

**Nutrition.gov**
www.nutrition.gov

**Organic Consumers Association**
6101 Cliff Estate Road
Little Marais, MN 55614
tel: (218) 226-4164
www.organicconsumers.org

## ORGANIZATIONS IN CANADA

**Canadian Celiac Association**
5170 Dixie Road, Suite 204
Mississauga, ON L4W 1E3
tel: (800) 363-7296
www.celiac.ca

**Canadian Diabetes Association**
15 Toronto Street
Suite 800
Toronto, ON M5C 2E3
tel: (800) BANTING
www.diabetes.ca

**Canadian Organic Growers**
125 South Knowlesville Road
Knowlesville, NB E7L 1B1
tel: (506) 375-7383
www.cog.ca

**The Canadian Society of Allergy and Clinical Immunology**
774 Echo Drive
Ottawa, ON K1S 5N8
tel: (613) 730-6272
www.csaci.medical.org

**Crohn's and Colitis Foundation of Canada**
60 St. Clair Avenue East
Suite 600
Toronto, ON M4T 1N5
tel: (800) 387-1479
www.ccfc.ca

**Dietitians of Canada**
480 University Avenue, Suite 604
Toronto, ON M5G 1V2
tel: (416) 596-0857
www.dietitians.ca

**Heart and Stroke Foundation of Canada**
222 Queen Street
Suite 1402
Ottawa, ON K1P 5V9
tel: (613) 569-4361
www.heartandstroke.ca

**Irritable Bowel Syndrome Association**
P.O. Box 94074
Toronto, ON M4N 3R1
www.ibsassociation.ca

**National Institute of Nutrition**
408 Queen Street, 3rd Floor
Ottawa, ON K1R 5A7
tel: (613) 235-3355
www.nin.ca

**Osteoporosis Society of Canada**
33 Laird Drive
Toronto, ON M4G 3S9
tel: (800) 463-6842
www.osteoporosis.ca

# Index

Page numbers in *italics* indicate recipes.

# About the author

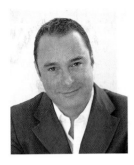

### Ian Marber
MBANT Dip ION

Nutrition consultant, author, broadcaster, and health journalist

Ian studied at London's renowned Institute for Optimum Nutrition, and now heads the Food Doctor clinic at Notting Hill, London. He contributes regularly to many of Britain's leading magazines and newspapers, including *Marie Claire, Eve, Attitude, The Times, Evening Standard,* and *ES*. In addition, he is an adviser and contributing editor for *Healthy* and *Here's Health*, two of Britain's most influential health magazines. Ian is also a sought-after guest on British television, appearing regularly on the BBC, Channel 4, ITN News, and GMTV, as well as on many radio shows. He has also made a 15-part series for the Discovery Health channel.

Undiagnosed food sensitivities in his twenties led to Ian's interest in nutrition. His condition was later identified as celiac disease, a lifelong intolerance to gluten. He is now an acknowledged expert on nutrition and digestion, and many of his clients are referred to his clinic by doctors and gastroenterologists.

Ian advises on all aspects of nutrition, and in particular on the impact that correct food choices can have on health. He is known by his clients to give highly motivational, positive, and practical advice that can make a real difference to their well-being.

His first book, *The Food Doctor*, was co-written with Vicki Edgson in 1999. To date, it has sold around 500,000 copies and has been translated into nine languages. Ian's first solo title, *The Food Doctor in the City*, published in 2000, highlighted how to stay healthy in an urban environment. It was followed in 2001 by *In Bed with The Food Doctor*, which examines how nutrition can improve your libido and help you sleep well.

In 2003, his book *The Food Doctor Diet* became an instant bestseller in Britain. Tested on Channel 4's *Richard and Judy* by three volunteers who each lost a dress size in only three weeks, *The Food Doctor Diet* has been hailed as a truly sensible, healthy approach to weight loss that actually works in both the long and short term.

# Acknowledgements

Thanks to all at DK for their enthusiasm, support, and food, especially MC, Stephanie, Jenny, Catherine, Hermione, and Antonia.

Heartfelt thanks to my dear family and wonderful friends and also to everyone at the Food Doctor. Special thanks to everyone who took the time to contact me with their success stories after reading and adopting the principles in *The Food Doctor Diet*.

The publisher would like to thank Zoe Moore for editorial assistance and Hilary Bird for the index.

# About The Food Doctor

Ian Marber and Vicki Edgson co-founded their Food Doctor nutrition practice in 1999 following the success of their original book, *The Food Doctor – Healing Foods for Mind and Body*.

The consultancy is now a leading provider of nutritional information and services, including a busy clinic in West London and a network of nutrition consultants operating throughout the UK. The Food Doctor offers one-to-one consultations, workshops, and lectures on a wide variety of subjects such as weight loss, children's nutrition, digestive health, and stress management. It also works with major corporate clients to improve the health and well-being of their employees and is frequently asked to work with professional caterers to ensure that a healthy choice of food is available.

The Food Doctor has developed its own food range to provide healthy meal solutions and snacks. All of these are designed to incorporate the Food Doctor ethos of balance and correct nutrition.